# Kicking
# Cancer
## to the Curb!

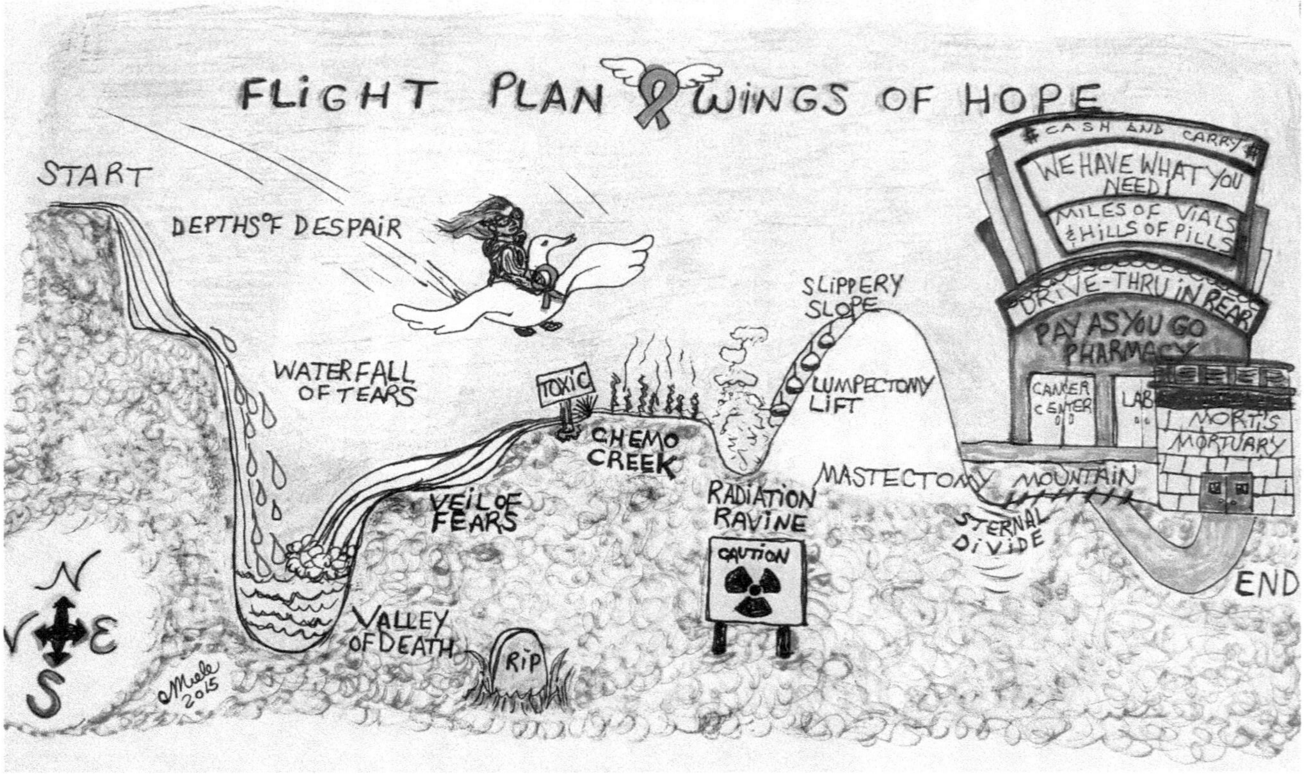
FLIGHT PLAN WINGS OF HOPE
START
DEPTHS OF DESPAIR
WATERFALL OF TEARS
VALLEY OF DEATH
RIP
VEIL OF FEARS
TOXIC
CHEMO CREEK
RADIATION RAVINE
CAUTION
SLIPPERY SLOPE
LUMPECTOMY LIFT
MASTECTOMY MOUNTAIN
STERNAL DIVIDE
$ CASH AND CARRY $
WE HAVE WHAT YOU NEED!
MILES OF VIALS & HILLS OF PILLS
DRIVE-THRU IN REAR
PAY AS YOU GO PHARMACY
CANCER CENTER
LAB
MORT'S MORTUARY
END
N
E
S
W
Miele 2015

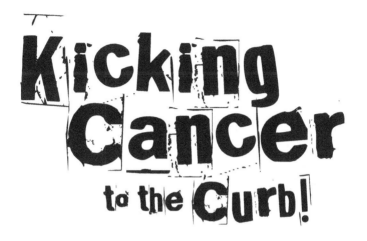

# Kicking Cancer to the Curb!

## A Glimpse of My Life as Seen in the Rearview Mirror and Through the Front Windshield!

**CAROL A. MIELE**

Paperback: 978-1-63767-136-8
eBook: 978-1-63767-137-5
Library of Congress Control Number: 2021904373

Ordering Information:

BookTrail Agency
8838 Sleepy Hollow Rd.
Kansas City, MO 64114

Printed in the United States of America

# CONTENTS

# DEDICATION

To my loving husband, Gene,
who spends all his nights close to me.
And to my loyal dog Flora,
who spends all her days close me.

# FOREWORD

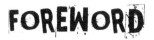

I t is an honor for me to introduce this second book by Carol Bruno Miele. I have known her for close to forty years and can say, candidly, that I have always seen her as strong and ambitious, but kind and gentle. She is a true fighter, literally kicking her demon, breast cancer, to the curb!

Reading her words, I was able to feel her pain and imagine her innermost emotions. And so will you as you read it. There are frank discussions of how the medical community, insurance providers, and your cancer have control over you. You will learn to overcome this, as Carol has, by taking the reins of your life and not letting cancer drag you down.

In the long haul, from diagnosis to her current treatment, Carol got through it all, but she was not alone. Her husband, Gene, was there with her every step of the way. She has often said that her first book, *Metastatic Madness*, was therapeutic for her. Allow this book to be therapeutic for you. Some of her poems will put tears in your eyes, while others will put a smile on your face. This is a book you will want to read again and again. Enjoy!

—Bruno J Panfili

# ACKNOWLEDGEMENTS

Chances are good this book would not have been written if it were not for the encouragement and support from my close friend and neighbor, Bruno Panfili. I would often hear him ask, "So, are you writing again?" or "When are you doing your next book?" I was *foot- dragging* because I didn't have the confidence in myself he did. After a time, I did write several poems that were swimming around in my brain.

I often have thoughts that pop up into my head anytime of the day or night. I hastily scribble them on paper and develop them later on. Occasionally, I'll fashion them into a poem or as part of an untold story. I experience a great emotional and mental catharsis after I write. It is a release and therefore, satisfying, much like the way one feels after a great meal or drinking a glass of vintage wine. I realized I still had a lot to say about my life, and my journey with cancer in particular. Without realizing it at the time, the second book had begun to take shape.

Much gratitude goes to my sister Dee Gillow. She has become a huge supporter who cheers me on. That last thought is ironic. Dee and I were three years apart in school, but we both were on the cheerleading squad in high school. We were selected to be co- captains of the squad in our respective senior years. I was happy to follow in her footsteps.

In reality, we were both naturals at giving the opponent a mouthful or two in the way of a loud cheer for our home team! Neither of us is known as having too few words to say . . . ever! Dee does a great job editing the first drafts of my poems. We have become closer since the onset of my cancer, and that's very comforting to me.

Another supporter I want to thank is Yvonne Panfili, my lifelong friend and the wife of Bruno. I call her my unofficial "Public Relations Rep" because she often has good ideas for promoting my book, or helpful critiques of my writing. We went to school together, nurses training, and later worked together in the operating room of a local hospital in Pennsylvania. We have been through the best of times and the worst of times, many of them together.

As it often happens in life, we went our separate ways in adulthood after we were married. She moved to Connecticut, and I lived in New York. We both came back to Pennsylvania eventually and now have come full circle as we are now next-door neighbors in Florida! We have shared many laughs over the years. We joke that it keeps us *young at heart*—may we keep that youthful laughter for a very long time!

As I've mentioned, my writing style is to jot down thoughts floating around in my mind. They tend to dominate my stream of consciousness until I get them on paper. Once written, I can move on to other things. After writing the fifth poem and a few pages of random thoughts on cancer, I realized Bruno was right. I decided to go ahead with another book. Once I did that, the thoughts flowed even more freely and easily, just like hot maple syrup and melted butter, running down over a stack of warm pancakes onto a large platter. Mmm, I love food references!

In my first book, *Metastatic Madness,* published in November 2012, I felt a more urgent emotional release. Writing that book was like having a dam burst forth and unleash all the pent-up emotion, fear, rage, and shock that I was feeling. It was my first ever diagnosis of cancer.

Shockingly, it was Stage 4 as it already traveled throughout my body, settling into my bones before I even had a clue. Looking back, I realize now why I had such backaches when I held my grandson Alex. He was just a few months old and weighed about twenty pounds.

After my husband Gene and I would spend a full day babysitting our grandson, my lower back ached for some time afterward, and I felt fatigued. I thought it was the effects of aging as we were now in our mid-sixties. My oldest daughter, Marisa, had just returned to her teaching job. We only babysat one day a week. With the backaches and fatigue, I wonder how I would have managed if she needed us more than that. I already had terminal cancer at the time but was totally unaware of it.

Slowly adjusting to the shock of having metastatic breast cancer, I wrote my first book. I wanted to share all I had learned in that first year and I desperately wanted to help others avoid some pitfalls. This is an incurable and life-threatening form of cancer; thus, it was an emotional upheaval for me, as it would be for anyone.

However, I was beating up on myself internally for not knowing or identifying it earlier on. I had just retired from a forty-five-year nursing career in which symptomatology, patient assessments, and critical thinking were drilled into us! How could I miss the symptoms? Easily, as it turns out, because, other than fatigue which I attributed to getting older, I had no actual symptoms.

At least, not until the day I had an itchy feeling in my left breast. It led to my finding the solid and rather large tumor that had been growing undisturbed and undetected for several years, despite a breast biopsy the previous year in the exact location of the tumor! It was reported as negative for cancer! Guess they missed it. *Very cunning, Mr. Cruel N. Cunning Cancer! You were missed on every single mammogram too!*

Having fibrocystic breasts since early adulthood, even my gynecologist found it difficult to examine me for signs of breast cancer due to my lumpy, bumpy, cyst-filled breasts. I did self-exams but never discovered anything solid. At least not until the itchy sensation led me to it. It turned out to be a lobular tumor which is long, spirally, and tough to find by means of palpation. It never presents as a round, pea-shaped lump, which is what we are always instructed to look for.

At the time, I was totally unsuspecting, and I wasn't aware of the implications of dense breast tissue (DBT), or that I even had DBT. No one had ever informed me. I couldn't advocate for further testing if I didn't know it should have been warranted. I have now learned so much I didn't know then, but it's too late for me to do anything about it.

So I pass these *golden nuggets* onto all of you, my astute readers, in hopes it will save you, or someone you know or love. Mammograms miss at least 50 percent of breast tumors in a DBT environment. Ultrasound or MRI testing is necessary afterward to identify the solid tumor growing in the white clouds that shroud it.

My first book, *Metastatic Madness*, had a dual purpose as it was therapeutic for me, and it was an effort to help others going through the same unfortunate situation I was experiencing. I hoped we would heal and recover together—a sisterhood and a brotherhood of tough but frightened cancer warriors.

Now, I hope that we are stronger and have left behind the side effects of chemo, radiation, or surgery, so we could forge new territory. We need to keep moving forward, to help others while helping ourselves. This synergy of our mets sisters and brothers will help to sustain us. We will use our combined energies to royally kick this cancer to the curb!

# A CONVERSATION WITH CANCER

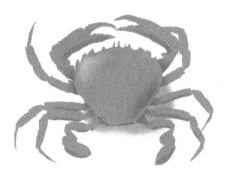

You have made the single biggest impact on my life, largely because you have the ability to take my life away from me. At first, you caused me many tearful days and sleepless nights. I was consumed with thoughts of losing all the things I love. . . my husband, Gene, my closest companion and pet dog Flora, my family, and my friends. Mostly, I will be saddened to leave behind my grandchildren. They are young, but so smart and full of life. I am crushed that I will not see them grow up. But there is comfort in knowing they are going to have bright and productive futures.

You have forced me to endure tests, procedures, and treatments that I never thought I'd undergo. I wouldn't wish chemotherapy on my worst enemy! But for you, it's largely just a delay tactic until you rally again and then seize your prey with a vengeance, to make your final deadly play. You are sneaky and wily, Cancer. You lay low until you have spread your disease-ridden, distorted cells everywhere, and then the damage is done! Often, by the time your unsuspecting prey is aware, nothing can be done to stop you or save their life.

You are also the worst kind of predator as you do not suffer from remorse or memory of your vicious serial attacks. Worse yet, you are a sniper who uses terrorist tactics. No sooner has a treatment been determined to be effective to stop you or slow you down, you change your colors just like a chameleon. You mutate into a different form that's resistant to the current treatment, leaving your prey helpless and hopeless! Possibly, there is another treatment option, but you know that time and good fortune is running out. You will, once again, be victorious!

You are the villain we can't take down, the heartless killer we can't incarcerate. Why do you continue to exist and threaten our lives? Why can't you be defeated? Cast off? Neutralized? Obliterated? Why are you able to outsmart, outlive, and outmaneuver even the brightest scientists, researchers, and oncologists everywhere? Are we destined to bow to your evil omnipotence forever?

"Yes," you say?? I think not!

# SECTION 1

# INTRODUCTION

Cancer lurked in my body for several years without my knowledge. It started in the left breast and eventually leaped over to the right one. It hung around long enough to wander through my bloodstream and seep into my bones. Once there, the cancer cells set up shop, eager to engorge themselves on unsuspecting prey—my *osseous* or bony tissue. The cancer ogre left the once smooth bones looking a bit more like Swiss cheese, with scar tissue that formed craters and holes. Not a pretty picture, or so I thought when peering curiously at my MRI.

Four months earlier, I had had laser surgery on my cervical spine, from C-3 to C-7. The orthopedic surgeon commented that despite the problems in my cervical spine which involved cervical stenosis, multiple *osteophytes* or bone spurs, foraminal narrowing, and two bulging disks, the rest of my spine looked like a train wreck. His exact words were, "It's a real mess."

Little did either of us know that I was already besieged with cancer cells. They traveled throughout my body, looking for places in which to nestle. Once in their new home, they nourished themselves in that microenvironment and multiplied. This process is known as *Stage 4* or *metastasis*, meaning it could be treated only to manage the symptoms and attempt to either slow it down or temporarily stop the metastatic process. A cure is not possible. It's fatal.

The cancer had metastasized to my thoracic, lumbar, and sacral vertebrae, as well as to my left scapula, sternum, pelvis, an area of ribs in the right rib cage, and the head of the right femur. Apparently, the orthopedic surgeon didn't have reason to suspect anything like that. After all, other than neck discomfort and increasing headaches, I was pretty healthy.

I do, however, recall the growing fatigue that would surface each work day around three in the afternoon. I would barely be able to stay awake for the drive home from work each day at four o'clock. I was feeling mesmerized by the road as the white lines whizzed past my front wheels. I recall leaving my driver-side window open for fresh air, even when it was freezing out, in order to remain alert.

I would also turn up the volume on the radio to stave off any stupor that might set in, as I caught myself nodding off a few times after being in a trancelike state. It was an increasing problem that helped me to begin seriously thinking of retirement by year's end. My husband was already retired and getting lonely at home all day by himself. I knew he wanted my company at home.

Combine that with my growing fatigue factor, gave me impetus to make the critical decision we all face after working an entire lifetime. Is this a good time to retire? Should I press on and work another year or two? Will we be financially stable and prepared for the long run if I stop working now? After working on our projected budget for the next year, I decided that if we scaled back to one car, we could afford my retirement.

As the New Year approached, I turned sixty-five years of age. I submitted retirement papers to human resources, spoke to the retirement counselor, and was cleaning out my files. It was a feeling of excitement and a great release of frustration that built up for quite a while over a failed promotion I was promised.

On January 1, 2010, I pulled the plug! I didn't have a large pension, but I felt our combined retirement incomes would be enough for us to live on once we sold our Mini Cooper sports car and Equinox SUV. We traded them in for a solid *all seasons* ride in the rugged Poconos of northeast Pennsylvania, a four-wheel drive Subaru.

I was asked by my *facility director* to put off retiring for a year or two as he was going to push through that promotion for me. This was the same promotion I had heard about for the past two years, the *director of quality and risk management*. I didn't believe him and saw it as a stalling technique, not meant for my advantage but for his. He had already assigned much of the director responsibilities to me. I couldn't refuse to do these assignments as it would be insubordination and there was no one else with my qualifications to complete them. I felt manipulated, patronized, and ultimately demoralized.

Sometimes, I think all the angst and the frustration that built up inside predisposed me to this cancer. Maybe not, but it sure didn't do me any good! I never looked back or regretted the decision to retire. When I learned I had advanced breast cancer ten months later, I realized, with great relief, that I made that choice timely. I wouldn't have to juggle chemotherapy and the accompanying debilitating effects along with a full-time job.

Soon after he retired, my husband, Gene, took over the task of preparing our evening meals. I was very grateful for that as I no longer had the energy to cook after a day's work. I had all I could do to just keep the car on the road during my sleepy commute home. He was a great cook and needed something to keep him occupied, so it worked. He had learned to cook at the hand of his father who was a butcher and owned the family-run business, *Miele Meat Market,* at 629 East 180th Street, the Bronx, New York. He had worked there along with his two brothers throughout their school years.

The customers would come in and ask how to prepare a roast or a particular cut of meat. With a little encouragement from the butcher and a healthy dose of confidence, they could pull it off and made the purchase. My husband would tell me in his best falsetto voice how they would besiege his father in those days, "Frank, how long I *gotta* cook the roast?"

Great tips and easy-to-understand instructions from the butcher and his helpers went a long way to sell roasts, chops, and steaks to these housewives. It also went a long way to move the inventory of meats and poultry the butcher stocked. You don't get that level of customer service in today's super-sized food markets. These new markets were the thrust behind the closure of many meat-cutting businesses. This particular line of work had been in the family for hundreds of years. Now, it is pretty much a bygone era.

Throughout his childhood, Gene had to toil away in the butcher shop after school and on Saturdays. All three sons were expected to work there; it was nonnegotiable. This expectation kept him from playing baseball or football after school with the

*CAROL A. MIELE*

varsity at Clinton De Witt High School. He had dreams of being a professional baseball player, just as I had dreams of becoming an artist or a writer. Neither of us got to do what we really had a passion for, but I'm fortunate that I have been able to realize my dreams on a smaller scale now that I'm retired and the cancer is stable.

If it's any consolation, Gene now has all the time in the world to watch sports, although, without a doubt, he would have preferred playing them when he was young, and savoring that memory now. He's a very loyal New York Yankees and New York Giants fan, even when they're having a bad season. He's also a racing fan. Sometimes he is watching a NASCAR race, a football game, and a baseball game all at one time!

It can make my head spin watching him click the remote back and forth. But he loves it, and I love him. We have learned to support each other's interests over time. He'll often say when I ask about us doing something or going somewhere, "Sure, if it makes you happy." Even if it wouldn't be his first or even his second choice, he'll go along with it to make me happy. We indulge each other, within reason, as do most spouses.

Cancer has changed our relationship in some ways. Gene has made my well-being the central focus of our lives. It has been out of necessity. I know that's not the way it is in all marriages. Many men abandon their wives after a terminal cancer diagnosis. It's true of breast cancer more so than other cancers. I suspect it has a lot to do with our culture and the tremendous value placed on women's breasts. Just think of all the breast implants and fashion designs that focus on an obsession with cleavage. Breasts are a hot commodity!

Of course, that's only if they're intact, healthy, and attractive. They may have suckled your young and brought a level of admiration or pleasure to your husband for years, but if you must have them surgically removed due to tumors that are spewing forth cancer cells, it can get ugly.

There are many women who have been left high and dry; stories abound of the so-called breadwinner who has left his cancer- stricken wife, along with the kids, the bills, and the mortgage. This is an American tragedy! How do you manage day to day with a life- threatening illness with no one to support you financially, physically, emotionally, or any other way?

After *Mr. Big* has gone, some women are unable to get the medication or treatment they require and have to settle for a substandard but affordable regimen. Perhaps society has placed way too much emphasis on our mammary glands as pure sexual organs. Despite the attractiveness of this physical trait, their primary purpose is to provide nutrition for our newborn. Any of you guys out there remember that?

Another area of total freaking unfairness and inequity is in the workplace. Women with metastatic breast cancer may as well have a scarlet number four on their foreheads. Once word gets to Human Resources, many go all out to *lay off* or *furlough* these workers. Apparently, employers don't want someone on board that may need time for chemo days or tests and not be there 100 percent of the time.

For many, this is the most crucial time to hang onto a job. Losing health-care benefits when you need them the most is demoralizing and can unravel even the most complacent person. Fortunately for me, my husband's health-care plan covered both of us. We have an annual $5,000 deductible. I never came close to reaching it before cancer. Now, we know we have to budget that amount each year. I would surely end up accumulating enough medical costs to reach that deductible before the year ran out.

Of course, just as you think you can manage a looming debt, someone comes along to raise the ceiling on it. Now, it's a $6,000 ceiling for family costs and $8,000 for catastrophic care. We expect it will keep inching up so that we are never quite able to make ends meet—a moving target. This is the reality for many people today.

Other than financial concerns, after my full recovery from a lumpectomy to remove the primary tumor, I realized my breasts were lopsided! The deficit was due to the large size of the tumor removed on the left. The tumor on the right disappeared completely with chemo, so that wasn't an issue. Although the larger one had shrunk 50 percent following chemo, it was still big enough to make a sizable dent after surgery. It wasn't all that noticeable to others, but it was to me. There's nothing like taking your bra off at night and find one breast suspended two inches lower than the other!

Also, the PET Scans were regularly reporting a mass in the left upper quadrant of the left breast. It was a toss-up: was it scar tissue from the lumpectomy or a recurrence of the lobular tumor? Not being a gambler, I didn't want to take chances. I wanted to know for sure which it was. Another concern was that I still had pain when lying on my right side. This was due to fibrocystic breast tissue I'd had for years that was predominantly on the right side.

With a breast reduction, I hoped to be rid of all these problems. My ample breasts were weighing me down and I looked forward to the lift this would give me! The breast reconstruction-plastic surgeon I met with made diagrams showing me where the incisions would be made. He was both informative and encouraging. It's certainly not a procedure for the faint of heart.

The yawning incision goes from the axillary line on one side of the chest, across and underneath the breasts, clear to the other side. Also, a vertical cut is made in the lower half of each breast, in the center line, up to and around each nipple. The undermining of deeper tissue can take place then. The remaining breast tissue and skin are deftly approximated to form much smaller breasts.

He explained that most of the tissue removed would come from the upper outer quadrant of the breast. Bingo! Good-bye to the dubious tissue mass resulting from the lumpectomy. He assured me that Pathology would analyze it thoroughly for cancer cells. The good news came not long afterward that it was *benign scar tissue*. Also, he was able to remove quite a bit of the severely dense fibrocystic tissue on the right that had bothered me for decades. I felt great relief about the positive report and losing all that nasty tissue. It was time to party!

I'd be remiss if I didn't say I like the compact, more attractive breasts he left me with. I went from a DD cup to a B+ cup and don't even need to wear a bra much of the time. I feel free after all these years of heavy-duty bras! Clothing fits better across the chest, so I'm no longer self-conscious and much more comfortable now in my own skin. I learned something else from my surgeon that's good news for anyone planning a breast reduction. Most breast cancers start in the upper outer quadrant. This is the precise tissue that will be removed in the breast reduction surgery. So a preventative effect is the added bonus as it will serve as a deterrent to breast cancer formation.

> *Turn your face to the sun and the shadows fall behind you.*
>
> —Maori Proverb

# Another Happy Ending

I need to write a happy ending,
It seems no one likes the real one.
It's not what people want to hear,
Because cancer's not much fun.

I could write another ending,
But I don't know how.
This life that I am living,
Is all that I know now.

If it were possible to do so,
I would obliterate all tumors.
So that every kind of cancer,
Would just be nasty rumors.

There'd be no need for pet scans,
No chronic joint or back pain,
No need for Cancer Centers,
Or this ongoing weight gain.

No flashing neon sign over my head,
Saying my days are numbered.
Just cancel all scans and injections,
And feel so unencumbered.

I'd be free to live my life,
Not sitting in the dark crying.
No need for constant treatment,
Or morbid thoughts of dying.

I'd have no telltale signs of chemo,
Like my embedded chest port.
I'd strip away all but my identity,
That would be a last resort.

I would ban all pink ribbons,
And any need to run a race.
No more ads promising a cure.
All cancer gone, without a trace.

The burning pain in my right hip,
And the one in my left shoulder,
Would be snuffed out like a candle,
I could actually think of getting older.

I'd put a moratorium on five year survival,
Die without the horror of predictions!
And the dubious longevity projections
No need for stages or other labels,

If only I could write a whole new ending,
I'd have no illness to make me queasy.
Nor would I have terminal cancer,
I just wish it were that easy.

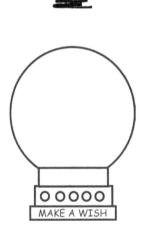

*In the room the women come and go, talking of
Michelangelo . . .*

*For I have known them all already, known them all:
Have known the evenings, mornings, afternoons,
I have measured out my life with coffee spoons.*

—T. S. Eliot, American Poet

# GAMBLING WITH OUR LIVES

L earning after the fact that my dense breast tissue (DBT) provided cloud cover for the breast tumors growing in both breasts was a huge shock! The density is largely fibrous tissue and completely occluded images of the breast cancer. According to my oncologist, the larger one on the left had been growing *a long time*. The biopsy showed it was *lobular carcinoma*. This is a slow-growing tumor. It was there long enough for the cancer to jump to the right breast. The biopsy showed the tumor on the right was *ductal carcinoma*, which is a more aggressive and a faster growing cancer. I'm thankful that it was detected early! I wasn't angry, but I was profoundly disappointed and disheartened to find myself in this situation.

I faithfully had had mammograms every year from forty years of age. That's twenty-five years of screening altogether, and no one ever told me I had dense breast tissue! They couldn't be truly sure if something was lurking inside. The tumors and DBT both appear as white clouds and cancel each other out. No one ever offered to do a follow-up ultrasound or MRI to see what might be inside those cloudy images. When I asked my breast surgeon why, in the case of DBT, follow-up tests aren't automatically ordered, she told me it's because "There are too many false positives. The insurance companies won't pay for them." I was taken aback! That's akin to throwing the bath water out with the baby.

Our very lives are at risk and the insurance providers have their eye on the bottom line. It's all about the money! I think *every* life matters. I think you can't put a price tag on any single life or play God and say who stays and who goes, who should get treatment and who shouldn't. It appears to me that many have, in fact, been sacrificed and offered up. I have had communication with a staggering number of women who, like me, were diagnosed with breast cancer for the *very first time* at Stage 4! That's inherently wrong! Too many of us are falling between the cracks!

Unless you live in a cave with no healthcare at your disposal, surely a cancerous tumor growing in your breast shouldn't go undetected by screening tests, at least not to the point that it has spread with wild abandonment throughout your entire body! I know of a number of women in their twenties and thirties that have Stage 4 breast cancer. They are the moms of little children and babies! They aren't even at an age when mammograms are allowed as a covered benefit. For anyone under the age of forty who wants screening for breast cancer via a mammogram, the reality is that no one will pay for it—it's on you!

Not having any screening caught these women I spoke of totally off guard. Some say they noticed a change in breast tissue, but had no inkling how serious it could be. They never dreamed their very life could be at risk. Some say they told their primary physician they thought something was wrong with their breast, but he had assured them it must be a cyst or some other benign tissue. After all, they were too young to worry about breast cancer. Not so!

We hear about screening and prevention all the time. What exactly is being done to screen and prevent breast cancer in women under forty years of age? Mammograms aren't done unless they ask for it, are willing to pay for it, and find someone who will order it. They are advised to do breast self-exams. These are critical, but how many women actually take it seriously and do it religiously, every single month? We have no idea of the compliance rate, as there is no way to collect accurate data on it. I suspect it's a low rate, especially with younger women who think they are invincible and not candidates for breast cancer.

But the most astute women I have talked with knew, without a doubt, there was something wrong in their breast. They learned of the changes through a breast self-exam and visual inspection. You know your body best! You know when something is different or changed from the recent past. But you'll have to convince your primary physician of that.

Many primary physicians do not know enough about detecting breast cancer and tend to rationalize it. They think you're too young or going through changes brought on by menopause or have cysts or other benign growth. Maybe they think you are manifesting hysteria and a paranoid obsession about breast cancer. You may feel doomed, until you find the right practitioner who will really listen to you.

I've talked with women who said their physician would not do any testing when they reported the abnormal breast findings. He simply didn't think there was anything to be concerned about. They had to shop around to finally find someone who wouldn't blow them off. By then, some were already metastasized! My advanced breast cancer was found by me while in the shower. So many years of mammograms that fell short through my entire adulthood. Now that's a waste of healthcare dollars! Not to mention the lives that hang in the balance, as mine does now.

Not very long ago, the Department of Health and Human Services proposed a change that would increase the age of the first mammogram to fifty years of age! Is anyone watching the store? This is tunnel vision at its finest and a rather callous approach to younger women. For starters, the younger the woman, the more aggressive the cancer is known to progress. Women over sixty-five are at greater risk because incidence increases with age. But these cancers, as a rule, are less aggressive and slower-growing. So if I am seeing this clearly, mammograms are targeted for the higher volume cases, not the higher risk cases. Something is radically wrong with that rationale! Isn't it time to stop the insanity?

> *The woods are lovely, dark and deep,*
> *But I have promises to keep,*
> *And miles to go before I sleep,*
> *And miles to go before I sleep.*

> —Robert Frost, American Poet

# Not the Long-suffering Kind

Dear lord, if I must be sick,
I just want to get over it quick!
Like when I had my tonsils out,
It was a pretty fast turnabout.

Swallowing anything was a disaster,
Full recovery couldn't come any faster!
Healing helped me to forget the pain,
Until it was time to have surgery again.

Cesarean-Sections aren't really so bad,
Went home with a baby and proud Dad.
The worst was when I had gall stone pain,
Thank God I won't go through that again!

The surgery was incredibly rough,
After that I felt I'd had enough.
The incision so long and so high,
I couldn't breathe, cough, or sigh.

My sister arrived on the scene,
She told me I was turning green.
But even that had a finite ending,
Six weeks and no deep bending.

So how did I end up with this disease?
One that has multiple locks and keys!
No one can open the mystery door,
It lurks and hides till it goes to war.

Unarmed, unaware, with no defense,
Against a monster without a moral sense.
You may find that medical help abounds,
You feel hopeful after twelve chemo rounds.

"It's going fine," I was reassured,
Despite the fact I can't be cured.
You've realized by now it's cancer,
The disease that has no answer.

"Not just any cancer!" I implore,
Why must I have Stage Four?
So much for total recovery,
It gamely ducks discovery.

We'll be in this union for a while,
I murmur with a bittersweet smile.
So I've learned to keep on truckin',
Make the best of what I'm stuck in.

Accept that no one's to blame,
In this horribly wicked game.
No quick turnaround here,
And no pink parades I fear.

But this time I'm in no hurry,
To get to the end, so I don't scurry.
Sit in the saddle and stay the course,
But I wish I was riding a different horse!

*Oh, my friend, it's not what they take away from you
that counts—it's what you do with what you have left.*

—Hubert Humphrey

# SECTION 3
# STATE DENSITY REPORTING LAWS

S ometimes it takes a *grassroots* effort to overcome protocols that lack the vision needed to provide comprehensive care. They tend to underserve us. This ultimately puts us in harm's way. For example, Nancy M. Cappello, PhD was diagnosed with Stage 3c breast cancer on February 3, 2004. This was just two months after receiving a *normal* report on her mammography. Less than 48 percent of women with Stage 3c breast cancer are alive after five years, so you can understand her strong desire to change the status quo.

She and her husband, Joe Cappello, set out to share the result of a decade of research about breast density with their local senator. This was after six physicians involved in her treatment refused to begin telling women the impact of dense breast tissue (DBT) on the validity and reliability of mammograms. They were successful in getting legislation enacted in her home state of Connecticut. Then, state by state, they plodded forward to get this legislation written to prevent delayed diagnosis of breast cancer.

In the past five years, they have gotten twenty-one states to pass this legislation. On February 4, 2015, a federal bill was introduced in the house and the senate. Dr. N. Cappello must be applauded for protecting us and for letting "the best kept secret" out, as stated on the website she established: *Are You Dense?* www.areyoudense. org. The new law mandates that anyone with DBT identified on a mammogram, must be informed of this by their radiologist. Once informed, an ultrasound or MRI must be done to more fully inspect the breast tissue for possible tumors or other abnormalities. The kicker is that the insurance company must cover the cost. Pretty comprehensive! !

What is it about DBT that this action had to be taken? Dense breast tissue, simply put, has less fat and more connective tissue. This fibrous, connective tissue appears white on a mammogram. Cancer also appears white on a mammogram. The end result is that tumors are often hidden behind the dense tissue. As a woman ages, her breasts usually become more fatty. However, if she should be unlucky enough to have a breast tumor start growing while she's young, she may not have the luxury of aging, or even getting to middle age.

Since 2010, there have been 36 states that have signed onto the Dense Breast Act They are: Alabama, Arizona, California, Conneticut, Colorado, Delaware, Florida, Georgia, Hawaii, Illinois, Iowa, Kentucky, Louisiana, Maryland, Massachussetts, Michigan, Minnesota, Mississippi, Missouri, New Jersey, New York, Nevada, North Carolina, Ohio, Oklahoma, Oregan, Pennsylvania, Rhode Island, South Carolina, Tennessee, Texas, Utah, Vermont, Virginia, Washington and Wisconsin.

While a mammogram detects 98% of cancers in women with fatty breasts,  it finds only 48% in women with the densest breasts.

In March 2019, the Department of Health and Human Services, the FDA announced changes to the MQSA (Mammography Quality Standards Act) to include reporting of dense breast tissue to the patient. Are You Dense Advocacy, Inc has been working on the proposed rule changes for over ten years.

During my period of chemotherapy, I received Medicare Summary Notices showing how much my insurance provider was being billed for my treatment. Each time, I would become nearly apoplectic. The high cost of treatment was shocking. With metastatic cancer, I will remain in treatment until I die. Before I have succumbed to this cancer, I will certainly have racked up a million or more in healthcare dollars. Multiply that by the high number of people living with Stage 4 cancer. Isn't that reason enough to prevent metastasis from occurring?

It's that simple, or that complex, depending on how you look at it. The way I look at it, I will cost the healthcare system and my pocketbook a lot of healthcare dollars. Add to that my co-pays and deductibles and my need for continuous monitoring and treatment. My mets will cost a great deal more than the *once and done* treatment of an early-stage breast cancer. Talk about wasteful spending. Let's put the money into prevention of metastasis rather than long-term, uber expensive treatment throughout and during the last stages of advanced illness.

If an ultrasound or MRI had been ordered after each one of my mammograms, my cancer would have been found at an earlier stage. True, it would be additional healthcare expenditure for the extra testing, but it would be a one-time charge for the calendar year. That's quite different than an unspecified lifetime of procedures, tests, scans, medication, repeat chemotherapy, and possibly further radiation, treatment, and surgery.

The latter is especially necessary in many invasive brain cancers where gamma knife procedures are used to dissect the tumors. Also, people with lung metastasis often require an insertion of chest tubes or other more invasive pulmonary procedures to rid them of excess pleural fluids or lung collapses. And the kicker is that my cancer could have been treated successfully at Stage 1, 2, or 3. In fact, following chemotherapy, radiation and/or surgery, I would just need an occasional follow-up. You do the math!

On second thought, you might not be able to do the math if you aren't familiar with these costs. Let me just tell you, my twice yearly PET scans cost four or five times more than an MRI. And they are quite a bit more than the cost of a simple ultrasound. My co-pay for a PET scan alone is $650 and they're done every six months to determine if my cancer is still in remission or if there is progression.

Progression means it's active again and I may need to have a medication change. There is a phrase you don't want to ever hear: "Your PET scan lit up like a Christmas tree!" The scan is like a heat-seeking missile looking for any cancer cells in the body. Actually, it is radioactive glucose (sugar) solution injected intravenously into your body about forty-five minutes before the scan is done.

A PET scan report of "no evidence of cancer" or NED would have images that appear bright green on the scan, whereas a "moderate amount of cancer cell activity", may appear yellow. Many cancer cells clustered together, as in a solid tumor, appear orangey or bright red. In summary, a finding of cancer looks like all the colors of a Christmas tree. You really don't want a holiday tree lighting up on your scan.

You want to be a picture of a calm, eco-friendly green. So doesn't it seem obscene that rather than allowing tests that cost a mere $100–$600 earlier on, this additional testing isn't routinely done until the cancer has actually spread throughout the entire body?

At that point, treatment will cost in the hundreds of thousands? It makes no sense at all! They are not only *penny wise and dollar foolish*, but also they are gambling with our lives. The healthcare system loses money, the patients lose money, everyone loses. Our friends and family lose us and we lose our lives. This is obscene when you think about it. Cancer sucks! And the protocols surrounding its screening, diagnosis, and treatment suck even worse. Fortunately for me, my most recent PET scan in January 2015 was NED or no evidence of disease. I'm good for another six months until the next scan—hooray!

There is a woman with bone mets that recently said she is on Medicare and it won't pay for costly PET scans. So she has to have CT scans coupled with a bone scan as an approved alternative. The combined cost of these tests is $2,000 more than a PET scan, a more efficacious test, would be. That makes no sense at all!

My faith in the medical community hasn't been totally shattered, but the third-party payers and their dogma is so entrenched that it dismays me at the very least. Their *less is better* mindset can be detrimental to our lives. So I have lost a lot of faith in the payers. Their mantra is *deny, deny*! How else can we explain all the young women dying before their children have their first or second birthday? Why isn't there a strategy to prevent a *first-time* cancer diagnosis that has already metastasized on a large scale?

Maybe we need to rethink calling those of us with Stage 4 *survivors* and get real about this— stop spinning outright lies about our illness! There is nothing we seem to be able to do about the *spin doctors* who want to make breast cancer appear to be a rosy situation. All we can do is hope the tales of an afterlife are true so we have something to look forward to. It reminds me of a song on the Rolling Stones album *Sticky Fingers* that's titled "Wild Horses."[1]

> *I know I dreamed you a sin and a lie*
> *I have my freedom but I don't have much time Faith*
> *has been broken, tears must be cried Let's do some*
> *living after we die.*

Sound too indignant? I think maybe not indignant enough! They do their best to have their way with us! We are admittedly over a barrel as we are totally dependent on reimbursement for treatment and costly medications. But give them an inch and they will take a foot. The survivor terminology is only the start. According to the American Cancer Society, a *survivor* is anyone who is still alive following a cancer diagnosis, even if that survival is only days, weeks, or months.

The term applies even if you are expected to die. Would they think of someone as a survivor of a boating accident if they fell into the ocean, got pulled out, but didn't recover despite several weeks in a hospital for care? Or receiving treatment for several months in a long-term facility? I don't think so. I think when that person dies, they will say he

---

1   Excerpt from "Wild Horses" by Mick Jagger and Keith Richards, The Rolling Stones, recorded in 1971.

never survived or he wasn't able to overcome the effects of near drowning after the accident.

Now, there is talk of declaring terminal cancer a chronic illness! Until they can cure me and only treat me for side effects and monitor me for the continued effectiveness of my long-term treatment, I prefer not to have my square peg put in that round hole! They want us to consider ourselves in the same category as people with diabetes, or other illnesses like it that require continuous monitoring and medication.

Really? Those people with true chronic illnesses could potentially die from them, but not necessarily so. If they are compliant and are treated properly, they may even die of natural causes or another illness entirely unrelated to their diabetes. I surely will not see that written on my death certificate. I'm certain of it. I feel that alone should exclude metastatic cancer from the long list of those illnesses characterized by their chronicity.

It might be an effort to take the pressure off the researchers who have not yet found the *Holy Grail* and cured cancer for all time. Or they are trying to brainwash us into thinking we are merrily rolling along, getting port flushes, occasional lab work and scans or other tests with nothing to write home about. How great it would be if Stage 4 cancers were just a matter of watching and waiting, all while enjoying life fully in between scans. Perish the thought—there is enough *scanxiety* to go around the world among *metsters*! We know that Stage 4 is 99 percent fatal.

Ask anyone who is Stage 4 and suffers from *the related anxiety* every time they wait for results of their most recent PET scan. It could feasibly come back reporting progression, or a cancer out of control. If you don't have alternative treatment options, you will likely succumb in weeks or months. We face our risk of dying all the time! I know many women who seemed to be doing fine and a month or so later, you hear they died. It's quite nerve-racking. That's not something you find in other chronic illnesses. I have other misgivings about this change in terminology.

At the risk of sounding paranoid, I am concerned that this shift to a chronic illness will signal an end to reimbursement for cancer treatment as we know it. Or an end to the freedom oncologists now have to do scans on a schedule of their choosing, or to select specific chemo agents to treat you with.

Chronic illnesses tend to fall into cookbook medicine where the entire treatment is set up in an algorithm carved in stone and very prescriptive for the treating physician, i.e., spelled out step by step. This is to save money by avoiding duplication, error in treatment, etc. But it takes away physician decision-making and troubleshooting. He might have to explain any deviation from it or the patient will be denied the treatment. Without it, you don't get to *pass go* or collect on the insurance reimbursement!

*The bustle in a house The morning after death*
*The sweeping up the heart, And putting love away.*

—Emily Dickinson, American Poet

# Crackled Glass

Just when you think you've got life figured out,
Along comes something to turn it inside out.

I had come to feel optimistic, that I had an edge,
But a cancer diagnosis put me out on a ledge.

I'm not ready to jump or to flee
My whole life flashes before me

Most of it chaotic disarray,
Like a kaleidoscope at play.

I'm frantically reaching for the Brass Ring,
Have a desperate need to latch onto something.

But that shiny, golden circle eludes me,
And holding onto my fears secludes me.

My broken parts had healed
My sadness all concealed

I was actually feeling stronger,
Felt I could last much longer.

Now it all seems hopeless,
Lost my compass, I'm aimless.

Cancer reared its ugly head,
Along with all I could ever dread.

Life can be unpredictable or a bore,
The Grim Reaper knocks on your door.

Then just as quickly slips away,
In its own inimitable way.

Some linger while others have perished,
Is it their DNA or were they so cherished?

Is it a powerful inner force not yet identified?
Something so mysterious it can't be verified.

I've heard tumors can shrink on hormonals,
Symptoms can actually go back to normal.

Then before drawing that last breath,
They're snatched from the jaws of death!

Healing occurs from the inside out,
Helped by the inner spirit, no doubt.

Deep inside is a fountain of glue,
It fuses broken parts like new.

The scars gently remind me,
My deep fears nearly blind me.

No longer pathetically torn apart,
My will fuels my beating heart!

My desire to live defies my Stage Four,
It's powerful enough to open the door.

That leads to the long-sought answer,
A cure for metastatic breast cancer.

Still I must question, where are the healers?
We are dependent on legal drug dealers.

Why do we still struggle with this disease?
Are we overrun by corporate thieves?

Meanwhile I exist like fragile, brittle glass,
Feeling vulnerable post removal of a mass.

This monster will return to threaten my life,
How do I sustain hope with all this strife?

# Expect Your Life to Change

Anyone who tells you they haven't changed after they have been diagnosed and treated for Stage 4 cancer are just fooling themselves. Not many other situations force you to revisit your life and reconsider where you've been, where you are now, and where you should be going. If you haven't done this yet, better get going! I'm not talking about geography here; I'm invoking cancer patients to reassess the totality of their lives. This reassessment includes:

- ✓ your lifestyle
- ✓ relationships
- ✓ daily activities
- ✓ long-term plans
- ✓ nutrition and hydration
- ✓ vacations or getaways
- ✓ savings and spending habits
- ✓ impact on your income and expenses
- ✓ pension plans and investments,
- ✓ smoking or alcohol consumption
- ✓ work status—if you are gainfully employed, the possibility of part-time work or early retirement

- ✓ daily activities and how leisure time is spent—you will have more of it and not feel up to a round of golf or a tennis match
- ✓ your religious affiliations or a lack thereof
- ✓ and many more facets of your life.
- ✓ Some or all of these will change!

You may be drawn closer to God or push him away. You may decide to dump a group of friends who have some bad habits that will no longer serve you well. You may end up divorced or jilted. You may be depressed and not want to be active socially, or you may long for the days when friends just dropped by and you could talk about anything without feeling there's a *white elephant* in the room. Changes will occur and you can't really plan for all of them.

I'm sure you've heard more than one cancer patient say, "You reprioritize your life." That's a pretty accurate statement. Often, people end up doing great things they were putting off for *someday*. Well, *someday* has just arrived, and that trip to Italy or Hawaii can no longer wait forever. Better get packing! But it goes without saying that you will need to take care of first things first.

If you don't already have one in place, see an attorney to get a *Last Will and Testament* drawn up. Another very important document is an *Advance Directive or Living Will*. You will need to assign a legal *Power of Attorney* or *proxy* for healthcare decisions. This is only activated if you are incapacitated. It means if you are unable to make the decision of whether or not you want extraordinary measures taken in the event your critical bodily functions are threatened, your POA will step in and speak for you in accordance with your wishes.

You may be in need of intensive medical care and support, like mechanical aids to maintain your respirations, heartbeat, brain, kidney, and liver functions. Death is imminent if any of the life-sustaining activities provided by these vital organs fail. I think you get the picture. This scenario is potentially the end of the road. So be prepared.

Most terminal patients opt for a *Do Not Resuscitate* or *No Code* order in such events. These days, not many people choose to remain in a basically vegetative state with feeding tubes, potent drugs, ventilators, infusions, and monitoring equipment that keep you alive and send out urgent alarms if that balance is threatened. When those alarms go off, the stampede begins. A crash cart, accompanied by a resuscitation team, arrives on the scene to do CPR and employs everything in their arsenal they can to reverse the cascading events that caused this medical crisis.

This team of experts will work to keep your heart beating. They will defibrillate it if it's beating too fast and ineffectively, unable to pump blood throughout your body. An intracardiac injection of epinephrine may be given to restart your heart if it has stopped beating. A temporary pacemaker may be attached to convert complete heart block to a life-sustaining regular rhythm.

They will intubate you if you are not already on a ventilator, and continued mechanical respiratory support will be employed to keep you alive. But are you really alive? Or are you a flesh-and-blood mannequin masked as a viable human being? You are no longer viable if you can't support your critical functions on your own any longer without these heroic measures. Is this your destiny? I hope not.

This is definitely *not* for me! I want to live, but I sure don't want to stagnate in an intensive care unit or other inpatient setting on artificial life support. I don't wish to obligate my family to visit a comatose body that was once me. It would no longer be me. It might look like me. Though I suspect, I would likely be bloated and have some contractures in my extremities, and so many tubes poking into or sticking out of every orifice that it would be disfiguring.

So I could be almost unrecognizable. It would be excruciating for everyone involved. At that point, no miracle is going to occur. That's your reality. You are on a slippery slope and in a moribund state. It's irreversible. If only you had opted for a calm, dignified death. If only they had allowed you to die with dignity.

It also leavesyouuopentoopportunisticinfections, skinbreakdowns, ulcers in the gastrointestinal tract, electrolyte imbalances, kidney shutdown, and bleeding or clotting abnormalities. There are a host of other horrific things that may occur that will not only run up your hospital medical bills beyond catastrophic, but toss you into that bin of hopeless cases. You will reach a point of no return. All this for the sake of someone not respecting you last wishes via your written healthcare proxy or a lack of having one in place.

It might be due to a family member who feels they must insist on having everything done that could possibly be done either because:

1.  they have guilt feelings arising from not doing more for you before all this happened, or

2.  they can't accept that you are going to die

Perhaps you have one of those physicians with a *hero complex* who can't let go as it might be seen as failure on his part. Or you have a physician with a *God complex* who can't accept defeat because he sees himself as omnipotent. This type of physician prides himself on having a low mortality rate among his hospitalized patients. It's a whole different thing if you die at home or even on your way to a doctor's office visit. But your death must not happen on his watch!

My cancer occurred over four years ago and I am still *alive and kicking*, as they say. I'm certainly well enough to write about it and to be a little snarky in the process. I am in remission and I am enjoying it! I've been given a second chance to do what I want to do with my life and whatever time I have left. When I asked the question, my oncologist was reluctant to give me a projection of my longevity.

She felt, and rightfully so, that it can be misleading and not apply to my particular case. When pressed, she told me three to five years longevity for advanced breast cancer. I've since learned that these statistics can be misleading as they are just averages and don't truly represent any one individual. She was right to be reluctant to give me the information I wanted. For some, it can cause them to be defeated from the start. For me, it just fired me up more to be the outlier, the one whose longevity isn't part of the norm or the average number.

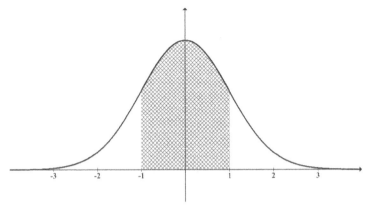

*Normal Distribution: Bell Curve*

If you're not familiar with *measures of central tendency* used by statisticians, the majority of people that fall under the bell curve are approximately 95 percent. They will live an average of three to five years after a diagnosis of Stage 4 cancer. The 2.5 percent that fall out of the curve and to the left of this normal distribution will likely live less than that, most likely two months to two years. Logically, the remaining 2.5 percent to the right of the curve would be expected to live longer than five years.

No one knows how long that might be. Some get to carve out their own longevity number as they are living longer than anyone projected. At four-plus years out, I'm hoping to be in that 2.5 percent of people who fall out of the curve on the right side of things. I intend to make the most of my time here on earth and wake up every day, happy to still be here. My work isn't done yet! Kick that to the curb, Cancer!

# The Cancer Dome

I'm living in the cancer dome,
It's the place I now call home.
People see me, touch me, feel me,
They try their best, but can't heal me.

My cancer journey is a one-way ticket,
Years of treatment, but I can't kick it.
It's Stage 4, that means it's metastatic,
Incurable and terminal, that's pretty drastic.

When I first landed here, I couldn't see,
Everything was dark and oh so lonely.
In time, I got to feel my way around,
My new domicile in Cancer Town.

There are many others, each in a dome,
"That doesn't make me feel better," I moan.
Sometimes I feel I'll run out of air,
Breathe slowly, don't panic or go there!

Pace yourself and learn to mark your time,
They gave me '3 to 5' like I committed a crime!
I want to break free, to go back home,
"Let me go!" I plead inside the cancer dome.

Alas, there is no exodus, no turning back,
So I've got a new plan of attack.
I'll look ahead instead, not back, only ahead,
But if that's all I do, I may as well be dead.

I need to fill my life with sunshine and flowers,
Get back to drawing, painting, and writing for hours.
So I called my Angels and got busy doing what I love,
Now a heavenly rainbow surrounds me above.

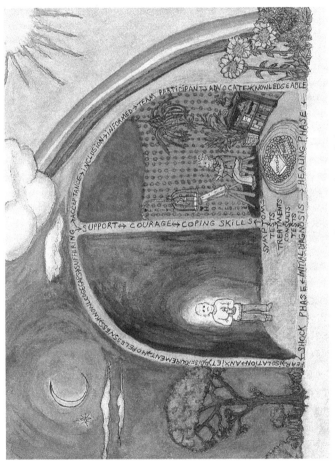

'Cancer Dome' by Carol A Miele

# THE ART OF CANCER

My maternal aunt, Rose, had breast cancer and underwent a radical mastectomy with excision of nodes on the opposite side that biopsied positive for cancer. This was in the early '70s prior to the new modified approaches to breast cancer surgery. The *slash-burn-poison* approach to cancer treatment as it's known by those of us receiving cancer surgery, radiation and chemotherapy is quite enough, thank you. But breast cancer surgery in prior decades was fairly extensive and mutilating.

The body disfigurement was a tough transition and recovery for women to make. There weren't modern techniques as we now have for breast reconstruction, like replacing breast tissue using full-thickness skin grafts from the abdomen and tissue expanders to gradually enlarge the breast size. No prosthesis needed in these new approaches.

Several years after this radical surgery, my aunt was diagnosed with metastasis to the bone marrow. It was unfortunate news considering she had already gone through so much and was raising her young daughter as a single mom. I went to her side for the surgery, a mastectomy, offering nursing care for the immediate postoperative period. I left her room for a coffee break on or about the third post-op day. When I returned, she was in the midst of turning her hospital mattress over and had stripped off all the sheets.

I believe I shrieked out loud, "OMG, what are you doing?" She replied that her mattress had a hole-like depression in the middle and she wasn't going to lie on it for one more minute! I suggested that she should have waited for my return and I would gladly have done it for her. It wouldn't have dawned on her that she shouldn't do this lifting by herself so soon after surgery. She was such an independent and determined woman.

She survived a total of thirty-three years with breast cancer, twenty-four of which were with metastatic breast cancer. That's an incredible record! Her team of hematologists and oncologists at George Washington University Hospital, Washington DC, often remarked, "Rose, your case is one for the books." She was a great role model of dignity and courage throughout her illness.

Rose was a competent woman of amazing strength, much of it arising out of the responsibilities she had in her job and those of raising her young daughter Karen on her own. Unfortunately, her final recurrence of cancer was discovered during surgery, when she had a hysterectomy in her late seventies. The pathology report showed the pelvic fluid to be filled with breast cancer cells. She died a relatively short time later in hospice. Despite her great fortitude, this monster finally wore her down. She was ready to let go.

When I think of her longevity, I feel that I would be very fortunate to have her genes. At least I know I'm not a carrier of the BRCA gene mutation. Cancer is hard enough without thinking that I'm passing it on directly to my daughters. And when I leave this earth, I hope to feel serene and peaceful, no regrets. I want to be ready to leave this life and transition into a glorious spiritual existence beyond this world as I know it. I also hope to be able to kick cancer permanently to the curb as my angels take me on a celestial journey, far away from the pain, far from the weakened, diseased state I will be in.

Of course, achieving that celestial state may depend on passing muster on *Judgment Day* to decide if I'm considered worthy enough to be admitted into heaven! I have my flaws, but they don't involve mass murder, pillaging, destruction of property, etc. Yeah, I know there's a whole range of sins I could be guilty of that fall outside of these examples. I am truly counting on the forgiving nature of the Almighty to overlook any previous sins or transgressions of which I may be guilty. I hope he's listening!

Throughout my childhood, I was always sketching or doodling. Known as one of the *artists* in my high school class, my high school yearbook refers to classmates browsing through my *art gallery* in a reading of the *class will*. I wasn't to achieve that level of professional artistry, but I have created some oil, pastel, acrylic, and watercolor paintings throughout the years, as well as charcoal and pencil sketches. It's a pleasurable hobby, not a career.

I sold some paintings when I was a young nurse just starting college courses for attainment of a Bachelor's Degree in Nursing. The money I raised helped pay for my tuition. Since my remission, I've enjoyed the return of a modicum of energy and motivation. Following the move to sunny Florida, I have really felt my creative juices flow. I hadn't created much since I was that young girl, fresh out of nursing school.

In the past year, I've done several paintings for friends and gifted them. I just enjoy creating something that gives them joy. Some have requested paintings of a beloved grandchild or pets that have passed on, current pets, or even portraits of themselves. I have been happy to comply, as it gives me something pleasurable to do. An added benefit is that it totally distracts me from thoughts of cancer.

Art is great therapy for cancer patients and a wonderful form of expression. When I'm painting, I am at peace and completely relaxed. Not being trained as an artist, I even hesitate to use the label of "artist" for myself, but I'm not sure what else you would call me. Maybe the label for me is *Outsider Artist*, a phrase my daughter Kristen introduced me to when she was in college studying fine arts. She did a project about my mother who liked to draw. It seems the *art gene* runs in our family.

She called my mother an *Untrained Visionary* and created a beautiful story about the drawings she did when both of my daughters were young and were sitting at her knee. Kristen studied *Outsider Art* at school. She said there are museums that collect this work and display them. We got to visit one of those displays of art at a museum in New York City. The artwork was by an elderly man who lived alone and created drawings over the years that no one knew about until he died.

As an untrained artist, I'm happy doing my own unique pieces on a small scale for a select group of friends who seem to love and appreciate them. I created a painting to donate to a local cancer wellness center. It was a pastel painting of Jesus carrying the cross down a winding road. He was followed by a throng of women with their IV poles hooked up to their ports for chemo infusion.

The tops of the poles look just like little crosses. I included young and old women and many diverse ethnicities. Some had bald heads, others had scarves or knit caps covering their baldness. The line of women goes on for as far as the eye can see.

The idea for this painting came to me one day during chemo. I would watch women trudging off to the bathroom, pushing their poles like they weighed a ton, their heads and shoulders sloped down as cancer fatigue set in. They would slowly shuffle across the floor. I felt great sympathy as I watched them. The cross formation on the IV poles struck me, and the concept for this painting was born.

I was pretty enthused about it and wanted to inspire women going through the horrors of cancer and its terrifying treatments. I wanted to assure them they are not alone and to tap into their spirituality to help them just get through this, one step at a time. I got it matted and framed and met with the founder of the cancer wellness center before one of my cancer center appointments, where she worked as a nurse.

She founded the center to honor her sister who died of lung cancer when she was a young woman. I was so impressed with her accomplishment. It's no easy feat. It's quite a beautiful place with offerings of individual or group education on cancer, support groups, massage therapy, and Reiki treatment for the caregiver as well.

I avoid the use of the term *cancer victim* if possible. Not because we aren't victimized by this dreadful disease, but because it's discouraging to think of yourself as a victim. It leads to feelings of powerlessness and hopelessness. I don't like giving in to that kind of feeling. It leads to fear, and fear is paralyzing at best.

There is another term I'm not comfortable with, as I discussed earlier. It's being referred to as a *survivor*. I don't feel much like a survivor. I have an illness that's terminal and is expected to kill me. It seems like the politically correct *cancer police* are putting words into our mouths. Not long ago, a survivor was someone who had chemo, radiation, and surgery, then was deemed *cured, free of cancer*. There was a magic number used in cancer circles. If you were still alive five years after treatment, you were golden! Now, those lines are blurred and these labels don't quite fit.

When I met the wellness center founder at the cancer center to give her the painting, I sensed she was disappointed as I uncovered it. All my excitement seemed so out of place now. Knowing that I'm not able to produce a professional rendering, I began to feel that's what she was expecting. I was actually apologetic when I handed it over to her. I was still hopeful, however, that in the spirit of doing the right thing, she would hang it in one of the waiting or meeting rooms at the wellness center so the women entering could see it.

It may not be great art, but it had a message I wanted to communicate. That did not happen. It remained in the bag on the floor of the front office of the center for some time. I'd see it there every time I went in. Feeling a pit in my stomach, I chalked it up to her busy life that just didn't allow her the time to hang it. Months went by and it never appeared. One day at the cancer center, I asked her where she finally hung the painting. She said it was hung in the business office.

That was a surprise! I asked her where that office was as I didn't recall seeing it and had been in all the places that visitors to the center are allowed. She told me, "It's a good place for it, as every new person who comes to the center goes in there and will see it." That didn't set well with me. I had never been in that office throughout the entire year I was going there. Also, it's a private office and not in the main part of the center where the other wall art is displayed. The one consolation I have is that the nurses at my cancer center saw it the day I brought it in for donation. They loved it! Some were moved to tears. They were all congratulating me on creating it. They asked for a color copy of it and hung it in the port flush/lab draw area where all patients who arrive are taken to get vital signs and weights.

Sometime later, a few nurses told me that it impressed many patients who came in and stopped to study it. So I did achieve my purpose but was sorry they didn't have the larger original painting to enjoy. I envision it sitting in a back room collecting dust.

This is where I confess that at a later date, I was at the wellness center and knocked on the door of that business office as I was curious to see my painting. No one was there and the door was unlocked. I knocked, then entered for a few seconds, scanned the room, and saw no sign of my painting. I closed the door and walked out.

I was crushed! I know her center is furnished beautifully and is very tasteful. Could she be an art snob? I decided she was. I just couldn't accept that someone would be so insensitive. I never went back to the wellness center because it made me feel sick to go there. And I never did another painting until my move to Florida where it all came together.

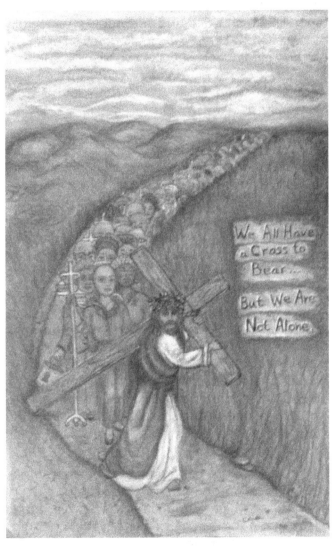

*'We Are Not Alone' by Carol A Miele*

Another change you might experience following a cancer diagnosis is the need to change your diet. In general, an anti-cancer diet includes nutrient-dense foods like fresh fruits and vegetables (especially the cruciferous kind), less meat, more fish and fowl, and the elimination of white bread, pasta, rice, or potatoes. Replace with healthier choices made from whole wheat, and use brown rice. Drink lots of water and eat fresh salads, nuts, and seeds.

The biggest offender of all is sugar! Don't ingest sugar as it fuels the tumors. Cancer likes sugar a lot! If you've ever had a PET Scan, a low carbohydrate diet is recommended the day before the test. You're given an IV infusion the day of the test with radioactive glucose— it's like a heat-seeking missile and will go straight to any cancerous tumors in your body. I use only naturally derived sweeteners like *stevia* or honey. Also agave syrup or monk sugar appears to be safe.

Because I'm on hormone blockers that cause joint and muscle aches and pains, I use turmeric powder daily. I simply sprinkle it on foods. It helps with arthritic pain as well. In addition, I use some supplements my oncologist suggested to decrease joint and muscle pain: glucosamine with chondroitin and MSM, fish oil, calcium with vitamin D3, and magnesium. I also drink tart cherry juice occasionally.

My tumors are estrogen- and progesterone-sensitive, so I'm on hormone blockers and avoid anything that might introduce or convert to estrogen in the body. For that reason, I avoid soy and soy products. I sometimes think about *Prempro,* the hormone replacement therapy I was prescribed when menopause started, bringing along with it hot flashes as natural estrogen waned in my body.

I read the literature quickly and noticed that it had a warning not to take the drug for more than six months. I asked the gynecologist treating me how long he recommended that I take it. He said in a nonchalant voice, "Until you're about ninety-six years old." Thank God I didn't listen to this insensitive clod!

Within two months of starting *Prempro*, I had cramping, backache, and vaginal bleeding. I stopped the drug immediately and found a plant source from red clover in a health food store. It's a phytoestrogen called *Premensil*. I took that instead. After about two weeks on it, I no longer had hot flashes and felt less irritable.

It's an over-the-counter drug, but it only cost me about $20 out of pocket for a one-month supply, and there were no side effects or precautions. A few months later, the report came out that *Prempro* was demonstrated in a controlled scientific study to cause heart attacks, blood clots, and breast cancer in women. Yikes! I think I may have dodged a bullet, or did I?

Some time ago, when I was in graduate school and taking a course on women's health issues, I remember we discussed a book called *Feminine Forever* by Dr. Robert A. Wilson. A best seller when it was published over forty years ago, the book helped persuade millions of physicians and their female patients that hormone replacement therapy (HRT) was not just helpful, but necessary.

His experimentation with estrogen employed research in an uncontrolled study of 304 women, ages forty to seventy, and was published in the *Journal of the American Medical Association* in 1962. These women were from a country outside the USA and knew little about experimental drugs. Since these weren't controlled studies, these volunteers took great risks with their lives and some lost out.

This physician author convinced women they didn't have to *dry up* and become *old hags* during menopause. He claimed that if they took this hormone replacement drug, they wouldn't have to experience hot flashes, night sweats, or anxiety. Their skin would be supple and glow with a slight pink flush, just like when they were young. In this era of innocence, not many questioned the claims of their doctors and wanted to believe the hype. I don't suppose any got to read this:

> "All post-menopausal women are castrates," Wilson wrote. "But, with HRT, a woman's breasts and genital organs will not shrivel. She will be much more pleasant to live with and will not become dull and unattractive."

Years later, progesterone was added to the mix and they were marketing HRT as the panacea for all menopausal women. Not many years ago, *Premarin* was the single drug most prescribed in America. The drug was processed from the urine of pregnant mares. After catheterizing these horses to remove the urine, some involuntarily aborted their fetuses. It was known to be a painful procedure to go through.

This information was shocking to me. Why create this risk for the mare and her unborn foal? Shouldn't there be a better way? And why is it that, in this country, menopause has become *medicalized,* made into an illness with its own unique set of symptoms and treatment? In other countries, it's a natural evolution in a woman's life.

In the Orient, women in Japan and China don't have hot flashes or any of the other *symptoms* of menopause. Some say it's due to their diet.

*CAROL A. MIELE*

Most women in the United States apparently have a negative view of menopause as a time of deterioration or decline in womanhood.

Women from some Asian cultures seem to have a different understanding of menopause. It's one that focuses on a sense of liberation, celebrating the freedom from the risk of pregnancy. Postmenopausal women of India can enter Hindu temples and participate in rituals, marking it as a celebration for reaching an age of wisdom and experience.

# On Getting Older

Losing bladder control at seventy?
Oh, how I wish I were just twenty.
My house is less clean and getting dirty,
Not the cleaning drive I had at thirty.

My body shape became portly,
When I rounded the bend at forty,
Retirement plans made me thrifty,
When I approached the age of fifty.

Off to those Golden Years I will go,
In the middle of the decade of 6.0
Maybe I should count back to ten,
And start this count all over again.

Got back to seventy much too fast!
And what about eighty—will I last?
No one categorically knows,
Not friends, surely not my foes.

Age is irrelevant anyway,
Your state of mind holds the sway.
I'm young at heart with a clever mind,
As I think ahead, and not behind!

# She's Got Everything! Yes, She's Got Cancer Too!

Know anyone annoyed by your every achievement?
Acting as though your success is to their detriment?

As though it was ripped right off their back!
And what you have is exactly what they lack!

I've had the misfortune of knowing,
Someone like that when I was growing.

She wasn't ever happy when I was "up",
Or the time I won the prized silver cup!

She would look at my life,
See a loving husband and wife.

"Oh! How lucky she is to be wed!
She'll never sleep alone in bed."

She would ogle my house and my car,
Act like I thought myself a movie star!

Not realizing I have a mortgage and loans,
Vet bills, cable TV and two cell phones!

I'm not privileged or wealthy,
And I'm not exactly healthy.

Outwardly, you'd never think,
My life could be gone in a blink.

That is the nature of cancer with "mets",
It's around long enough to rack up big debts.

You worry if unfinished business is closed out,
Having a terminal condition gives you no clout!

"Well, I just thought she had everything!
A house, a husband, and shiny gold ring.

Who knew she was hocked up to her neck?
Guess cancer bills made her life a wreck!"

"I wasn't aware she was so sick she could die!
Thought she had whatever money could buy."

But a cure for cancer can't be bought,
Nor is it a matter of how hard she fought.

Their estimates of you are worthless,
They never look beneath the surface.

Not interested in what's below the skin,
Unaware your true value lies within.

Her eulogy won't be about possessions,
Or long held casual impressions.

In life, she lost as much as she gained,
She soldiered on despite feeling drained.

Willing to work for whatever she sought,
Braving the scars from the battles she fought.

She had most everything she ever wanted!
With supportive love, she felt undaunted.

A woman who seems to have everything,
Is quite often harboring something.

It could be an ancient family scandal,
Or hard-earned money mishandled.

We all have skeletons in our closets,
Maybe someone made a bad deposit.

The bank policies could be so cruel,
You feel like you're back in school.

I seem to live in a house made of glass,
My medical history is seen en masse.

So why is there all this speculation?
I've been made into their own creation.

Oh, that I could be what they've conjured,
Instead of cancer-stricken and bone-injured!

*Throughout the centuries the sufferer from this
disease has been the subject of almost every
conceivable form of experimentation. Hardly any
animal has escaped making its contribution.*

—William Bainbridge, American Military Hero

# ESCAPE TO PARADISE

After much deep thought and some hand-wringing, my husband and I made the move to sunny Florida to escape the cold, bitter winters of the northeast. We lived in the Pocono Mountains of Pennsylvania, known for their ski slopes and year-round resorts. They have many recreational winter sports to offer, like snowmobiles, horse-drawn sleigh rides, ice skating, snowboarding, toboggans, and of course, skiing, both cross-country and downhill.

However, an environment suited for these winter sports also has a downside, such as the icy and treacherous roads, deep freeze temperatures, record-breaking snowfalls, and all the risks associated with those weather conditions. I'm sorry to say that I have had firsthand experience with some of the worst storms to hit the Poconos and the northeast region of Pennsylvania during my commutes to and from work.

The most harrowing of these occurred in March 1982 when I was a staff nurse working at a veterans administration hospital in northeast PA. On the best of days, it was an hour-long commute. In the scene that follows, you will see how that could end up being caught in a nerve- racking five-hour struggle to get home in an ice storm.

I worked the second shift from 4:00 p.m. to 12:00 midnight for a period of twelve years so we could manage child care. We had no day care nearby, so my husband worked daytime hours. I worked at night. I was a sitting duck when a storm hit during my working hours. Traveling at night up mountainous country roads with no gas stations or emergency services is risky business. One particular storm occurred when I was five months pregnant with my second child. My older daughter, Marisa, was only seventeen months old at the time.

Trying to keep a watch on the weather as my shift progressed, I heard there were quite a few accidents on Route 81, a route that led to my parents' home in Old Forge. There were eighteen-wheelers lying in the roadway and the highway was closed for miles. That cancelled out my emergency plan to stay at my parents overnight rather than take the risk of driving all the way up the mountain to the Poconos in the midst of this storm.

With no alternative, I left work shortly after midnight and managed to hold the road pretty well in my four-wheel drive vehicle most of the way home. I was feeling pretty confident as I saw many cars along the way that had slipped off the road and were lying in ditches. I just kept telling myself to go at a steady pace and keep moving forward. No sudden braking or turns or other quick changes in speed or direction and I would eventually get home.

Of course, the usual one-hour drive took me three hours just to get to the entrance into my community Indian Mountain Lakes. I was so grateful to get this far, I didn't care how long it took. I was now just a little over a mile from the warmth of my home, so I relaxed somewhat. Little did I know that my nightmare was just beginning!

No sooner had I driven through the entrance to my community, I noticed the road surface had changed from a slippery though manageable snowy cover to a slick, icy wet surface. As I began the slight uphill climb on Scenic Drive, I observed that the snowfall had turned to mixed precipitation. That created thick fog along with sleet and icy rain. The rain had washed away the cinders that were put down earlier on the road surface.

It was now 3:00 a.m. and absolutely no one was on the road. Everyone was safely tucked away in their beds except me, the pregnant nurse who was trying to steel her nerves and not freak out! It was totally silent now. You could hear a pin drop, or in this case, icy rain drops. As I proceeded forward, I slowed down to less than ten miles per hour because I couldn't see beyond my headlights any more.

The rain had started coming down harder and my car began to drift. I was losing traction on the road surface. As the crest of the hill was approaching, I decided to steer my car over to the right, just enough to get two wheels on the shoulder for more traction. That move helped me get to the top of the hill. Stopping the car to assess my next move, I tried to survey the road ahead as well as I could because now I had to face going downhill.

It wasn't very helpful for me that I have a fear of heights. That hill was a lot scarier in the midst of an ice storm. It was especially so knowing that I had to make a right turn in the middle of the hill's incline to access the road leading to my house. That thought left me physically shaky. I'd never make that turn on this ice. I would end up in a ravine in the woods, if I was lucky. Worst-case scenario would be sliding down the entire hill backward till the car slammed into something, then being trapped inside with no one to rescue me.

My heart began to pound and my pulse quickened. I was becoming quite alarmed as my previous confident stance dissipated into the icy, dark, thick fog of the night. This was a whole new set of circumstances. I was more worried about preserving the safety of my baby than anything. I slowly inched the car forward, only to discover that it was unable to hold the road at all.

The wheels were behaving as though they were independent of my steering wheel. I felt as though I was navigating a boat when my vehicle slid slowly to the left, then to the right. I had a flash visual of the wheels not even touching the road surface because they were floating on a surface of ice water coating the road.

This caused me to nearly lose my nerve! I made my best attempt to remain calm and move the car further so it sat on the right shoulder of the road. I did what I could to get it off the road. The road surface was definitely not suitable for driving, unless you fancied sledding downhill like grease lightning.

Once on the shoulder, I got out and saw that I was partially submerged into thick crunchy snow to the right, in the midst of branches, small trees, and shrubs. The car wheels were on a rough but icy surface. I couldn't see any further than right in front of my feet. That was when I decided to abandon the car!

I had pretty much lost all orientation as the fog surrounded me like a thick blanket. I walked around from the driver's side to the front of the car, holding onto anything I could grasp. The only sound was that of the icy rain hitting the road surface, not very comforting. Of course, I knew I wasn't going to see a plow truck or emergency vehicle in the midst of this ice storm. I inched my way further right to the berm of the road.

I sensed that I was there when my feet stopped sliding on smooth ice and, instead, made a crunching sound as they sunk into the icy crust that formed over the snow. I had on a winter down parka, but underneath was only my thin white nurse's uniform, stockings, and work shoes. The shoes had a smooth rubbery sole and heels to cushion tired feet that were mostly standing on a busy shift. They were not designed for gripping wet and slippery surfaces and were definitely not winter footwear!

Walking on the berm of the road gave me the advantage of holding onto trees and branches to steady myself. I began to feel that I was moving in a declining direction and braced myself for the downhill trek. I made it to the corner and turned right. Now I had only two blocks to walk to get to my house. Unfortunately, halfway there, I had to walk through a huge puddle of ice water that completely submerged that part of the road.

I didn't realize how deep the water was until it seeped into my shoes, completely soaking my feet. That was a further shock to my system. My parka had a fur-trimmed hood that now looked like a dead animal hanging off my shoulders. It was soaking wet. I was getting drenched with very cold water that soaked through my thin nursing uniform as the rain continued. Could this night truly get any worse? Well, yes, it could.

There was no time to take it all in and feel sorry for myself. It had taken me nearly an hour to trudge through a mile of ice- and water- covered road to avoid a fall. I was forced to take baby steps to avoid sliding. Thinking of my steep 185-foot downhill driveway, I realized I still had the worst part of my trip to go and was running low on energy.

Finally, I reached my house and was standing at the top of the driveway. It was a beautiful sight! The fog had lifted enough for me to see the glistening ice surface with the moon's light reflected off it. It was smooth and shiny, nature at its finest and at its most treacherous.

There was no doubt in my mind that I couldn't possibly survive walking down the sheer drop of the driveway. I opted for going downhill in a sitting position. Standing erect was no longer feasible. I sat down on the side of the driveway on a soaking wet uniform that provided no protection from the freezing cold, wet surface.

Sliding down the driveway, I grasped any branches I could to slow myself down as I began to pick up speed quickly. When I reached the bottom, I prayed and thanked God for getting me this far. The last leg of this arctic adventure was not going to be the kindest part by far. It was worse than I could have imagined!

I couldn't stand up when I reached the bottom of the driveway. The ice was bumpy and full of deep ridges that I couldn't tread. It looked strangely like an ocean that froze in place with deep ribbons of waves coming to shore. I suppose it was from the harsh wind. No longer being on a steep incline, I couldn't slide toward the house. I only had one choice. I got onto my hands and knees, then crawled on all fours like some animal on the prowl.

That was when I realized I didn't have the remote garage door opener with me! I had left it in the car. The garage was beneath the main floor of the house. Without the garage door opener, I had to navigate the full set of steps leading up the deck to the front entrance door. The set of sliding glass doors in the basement level were bolt locked. No key was going to open them. As I got closer to the steps, I gasped in horror!

The banisters and steps were covered with approximately two inches of clear ice. There were also thick icicles hanging from the banisters that were at least two feet in length. I had nothing safe to hold onto. The house was in complete darkness. My husband had fallen asleep after waiting hours for me to return home. It was now after four o'clock in the morning. I snapped off some icicles and threw them up at the deck windows. I hoped to make enough noise to wake him up.

It wasn't long before I realized my efforts were futile. Unlike rocks, the icicles just glanced off the icy surface of the screen covering the windows. They fell back to the ground almost silently. Our bedroom was in the back of the house, so he would not have heard me unless the noise was the equivalent of a small bomb going off. I was fresh out of luck. Only thoughts of my unborn child gave me the sheer will to scale the steps.

Shaking from the cold and wet clothing, the fatigue, and the fear of what all this cold and stress might be doing to my baby, I confronted the danger now facing me. I very slowly began my ascent on my knees. Those thirteen steps seemed more like climbing Mount Everest to me. Placing my shaking knees one at a time onto the ice-covered steps was totally unnerving. I held onto the step above me to get some leverage by wrapping my arms around. Then I slowly raised myself enough to reach the next level.

I repeated this, step by step, until I reached the top. Each time I moved upward, I prayed I wouldn't slip and fall downward. I didn't feel I had the energy reserve to repeat this arduous exercise, assuming I would survive the fall well enough to climb again. God was with me that night. He must have been, as I have no idea where I got the fortitude to see this through and make it to the top.

When I reached the deck landing, I could barely stand up because I was shaking so much. My legs felt like rubber. I inched forward, trying my best to balance myself and not fall when I was so close to safety. It was about six feet to the door, a dozen or so baby steps to get there. As soon as I got inside, I just fell into a heap in a chair and the tears began to fill my eyes.

My husband awoke to my crying and came into the room in shock. I was a sobbing and heaving wet mess, fueled by the hormones of pregnancy and the stress of a traumatic and prolonged crisis. I looked like a wet rabbit who escaped sudden death from a predator within just a hair of its life.

Gene helped me pull off my wet clothing and get into dry warm nightclothes. I drank the warm tea he made, and when my sobbing had stopped and I was calm enough, I crawled into bed and collapsed into a much needed night's sleep. It was nearly five o'clock in the morning. I had left work at midnight. What a nightmare!

Fast forward to the present and where we live now, in *Paradise*. That's what I like to call it, because it truly feels that way. North central Florida is a pretty cool place to be. You can travel east or west for one to two hours to get to the ocean and the very best beaches available anywhere. You can travel one-and-half hours south to visit Disney World or any of the many places that offer fun for all ages in the Orlando, Miami, and Tampa vicinities.

You can travel north for less than an hour to visit some of the finest horse farms and specimens of great thoroughbreds to be found anywhere in our country. Ocala is known as the *Horse Capital of the World*, and for good reason. They have bred and raised a number of famous championship horses, including *Affirmed*, the last *Triple Crown winner*. Or you can stay right here in Ocala for all the fine things it has to offer, including great restaurants, live theatre, art museums, shopping, and many parks boasting the finest fresh water springs found anywhere.

We are so fortunate to make this move before my cancer advances. We'll be able to enjoy our lives now while we're still active. The warm climate and access to many venues we're attracted to, makes it very easy to put together a quick getaway. We are like kids again, excited to see new places and curious about the coastal environment of the communities strung all along the eastern and western shores of Florida. We ditched the four-wheel drive vehicle and got a red convertible so we could truly take advantage of sunny Florida and the scenic sites it had to offer.

Our favorite place for fun in the sun and a totally laid-back feeling is Key West. We'll be going back there soon for a brief visit. Hopefully, we'll get to the *Schooner Wharf Bar*. It's an outdoor, open-air bar right on the docks. You can watch the tall ships come and go, see the spectacular sunset that makes Key West so unique and so special. We can enjoy the balmy breezes, noshing on fresh shrimp and sipping on a cool tall one or a frozen Margarita. Yes, this is what we call living! Cancer, I'm going to kick you to the curb—you are in my way!

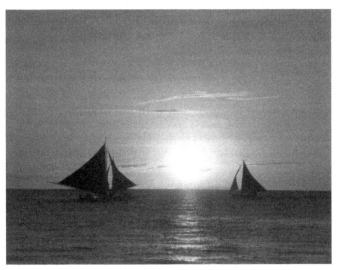

*The brave may not live forever, but
the cautious don't live at all!*

# Strong in All the Broken Places

This poem was inspired by the words of Ernest Hemingway. In *A Farewell to Arms*, he wrote, "The world breaks every one and, afterward, many are strong at the broken places." Not everyone becomes strong though. Some remain broken. Some of us are more resilient than others. Some people have already had many burdens in this life, and this was just one too many. For others, it becomes the greatest test of their will.

I've had my share of broken plates
and other fragile things.
Mending them with glue, I'd hope
the scars would not show.
No matter how careful I was after my meticulous repair,
It eventually broke again and in the trash it would go!

The integrity is gone; it's weakest where broken,
It won't ever be new again, not even next-to-new.
The glued cracks and scars will snap wide open,
Must handle with care and watch what I do.

So what of broken humans who fall apart?
Do they fare better or much worse by far?
Like the jagged seams of my last catastrophe,
Could a human overcome that ragged scar?

Pondering our heroic military figures in history,
Fighting battles both near at home and afar.
Did they recuperate from scars on the outside?
How much healing took place beneath the scar?

Some may die of old age and vaguely recall the fear,
While others may be hopelessly fused to the trauma.
Shadows loom over them at night to disturb their sleep,
Explosions go off in their heads as they relive the drama.

*CAROL A. MIELE*

The scars of cancer also run very deep,
Emotionally you just can't get away.
It's a nightmare deep within your psyche,
You just might as well stay.

Though you're on borrowed time,
You distract yourself and hide it well.
But those who truly know the real you,
Are aware you're in a living hell!

Before long, I felt I could not accept that fate,
I climbed out of the dark hole and broke free.
Though I struggled, I soon regained my stride,
Surging forth to face life's darkest mystery.

I believe in the adage I have heard many times,
"What doesn't kill you makes you stronger."
Cancer has broken me in so many ways
But it doesn't control my spirit any longer.

I've stepped away from all the grief and worry,
Living each day with people and things I love.
I don't look back or think about tomorrow,
I'll live in peace till the Angels call from above.

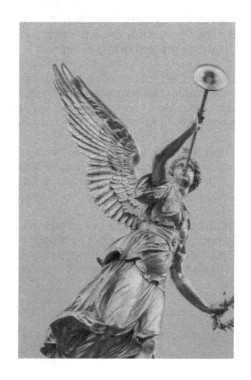

*Whoever said winning isn't everything,*
*obviously wasn't fighting breast cancer.*

—Author Unknown

*CAROL A. MIELE*

# SECTION 7

# HOW MY LIFE CHANGED

Life after chemotherapy isn't exactly an afterlife, but you could have fooled me. So much has changed in my life after my diagnosis and treatment that I feel like I'm living a different life. I have lost the *old me* and have worked very hard to embrace the *new me*. You might be asking yourself what those differences are.

In many cases, women who have had mastectomies, with or without plastic surgery or reconstruction, have a lot of changes to deal with externally. I'm sure their internal differences feel insurmountable. Not having to deal with disfiguring surgery except a *lumpectomy* to remove the primary tumor, most of my changes were internal. Some were buried so deep in my psyche that I still can't get in touch with them!

The *old me* saw the world differently. That feeling was borne of a sense that I would go on for a very long time and die of natural causes at a ripe old age. I innately knew that I had many more great experiences ahead of me. I just had to pick them, like ripe shiny red apples on a tree, and snatch them away for my pleasure.

I thought the world held infinite possibilities for me and my family! We didn't have a lot of cash flow when I retired. I had retired the same year when I was hit by the *Cancer Depth Charge*, which left me with many medical expenses. But if we had enough interest in a destination, we would work out a practical travel plan that would allow for a fun vacation.

There also would be many more birthdays, anniversaries, holidays, Christmases, and adventures ahead of me. I relished each and every one, mostly because they brought our family together. At this point in our lives, our daughters were living independently and had busy lives. So these family affairs held special delight for me. As you can see, my mind was loaded with forward thinking and joyful anticipation of future events.

Most of the changes the *new me* experienced since diagnosis were in the spiritual, psychological, and emotional spheres. I haven't experienced many physical changes because it's advanced breast cancer. A mastectomy isn't recommended and wouldn't have helped me. I was beyond a cure and, as someone not so graciously put it, *Once the horse is already out of the barn* . . .

Once you've metastasized, there's no benefit to having the breasts removed." My oncologist explained that my options were chemotherapy and a lumpectomy after I went into remission. There was no indication for radiation. I felt relieved after the primary tumor was removed. It was a tremendous psychological lift. I wanted that *bad boy* out of there! It was like a bomb buried inside me that would go off someday and take my life with it. I wanted it *out*!

# The Killer Within

Not so very long ago,
I came to intimately know
A killer who lives within
No, I didn't let him in.

I never heard a knock.
It was such a shock!
All at once he was there,
Now life hangs in thin air.

He's taken away so much,
I cringe to his very touch.
Just knowing that he's near,
Draws me into a state of fear.

Fearless, cruel and cold,
He's killed before, I'm told.
Its certain he'll kill again,
It matters not who or when.

He'll go on a rampage one day,
Still, they haven't put him away.
Lock him up, throw away the key!
Show him not one bit of mercy!

A life sentence is not enough,
There's no punishment too rough.
Use any means to slay the beast,
Leave his corpse for prey to feast.

He's been a plague to all mankind,
Don't leave a bit of trace behind.
Show him we finally have the answer,
To destroy the monster we call Cancer.

*Do not go gentle into that good night,*
*Old age should burn and rave at close of day;*
*Rage, rage against the dying of the light.*
*Though wise men at their end know dark is right.*

—Dylan Thomas, Welsh Poet

*CAROL A. MIELE*

# SECTION 8
# SPIRITUAL CHANGES

rarely looked back, especially if it was a painful experience. The past was just that, it was gone. But the *new* me post-cancer treatment seemed somehow riveted to the past, especially the memory of my parents, who are both deceased. I think many cancer patients get sentimental and long for a time when they were healthy, happy, and younger—when they had not a care in the world!

I longed for the comfort and security of being healthy and in the care of my parents, rather than being terminally ill with a team of specialists. How good it would feel to have my parents wrap their arms around me and console me. I needed them to tell me that I will get through this just fine. They always saw me as a strong person, a go-getter. I need to be reminded of that part of me now, because this terminal cancer has frightened me to the core!

This doesn't in any way negate the support and nurturing from my husband, my children, close friends, or other family members. But they aren't my Mom and Dad—the two people knew me from birth and placed me under the Christmas tree. I was born on Christmas Day in 1944. I was wrapped in a baby blanket, swaddled like the baby Jesus, when they got home from the hospital on New Year's Eve. As a child, I loved hearing that story! I enjoyed bringing them any amount of joy as I grew up. I loved them wholeheartedly, despite any flaws, disappointments, or shortcomings, and always will.

I also felt a desperate need to reach up to someone older, stronger, and wiser. I wanted to connect with the two people who knew every kink in my armor, every quirk or hang-up, people who knew who I really am. They would know what to say and how this terminal illness is affecting me. My parents were the only two people who witnessed all of my early-life experiences. These experiences shaped me and made me the woman I am today.

While I was shaped by many other factors influencing my life, this is the single most important one—the imprint left by my parents. I often think I didn't really learn who I was and have a good sense of self until I was thirty years of age. But I do know that those rudimentary building blocks, upon which my foundation rests, go right back to my mother and father.

I longed for that unconditional love, that arm around me telling me everything will be okay. No matter how old you get, your spirit sags a bit more when you have no parents around to beam proudly at your accomplishments or help relieve you of your suffering when illness or tragedy befalls you. Your spouse and/or children can fill that need to a great extent, but it's not quite the same thing. You have more history with your parents.

I also think it goes back to our vulnerability in childhood. I have a vivid, singular memory of being carried by my mother on a cold night to visit my grandfather. It was a three-block walk. The sky was inky dark and dotted with bright stars. It was so clear that night, I could see little puffs of breath coming from my mother's lips as she carried me.

I could hear her breathing and her strong heartbeat. It gave me such a sense of security. I felt that we were one. This feeling of belonging, love, and security in the mother-child bond is priceless. If you're lucky, that feeling will follow you and bathe you in its warmth for a lifetime.

My parents—there was no one else who could fit that description or that need for nurturing. All of my close aunts and uncles were now deceased and my sister was too close to me in age with a three-year gap. She would remember a lot of my early days but is too young to know the earliest years. These were the years in which my confidence and sense of self took shape. I was at an impasse, one marked by longing and needing.

Then the realization came to me one day that since my parents are no longer with me, I might be able to fill this need for comfort and security by reaching out to God, the Heavenly Father. Who better to turn to? Who loves us more and is more invested in us but the one who created us?

Why didn't I think of God before? Isn't he the only true one that knows all of us—intimately? Isn't he the Savior that all hopeless people go to for even an ounce of hope or courage or for a just a smidge of reassurance and a little nudge in the right direction? Would he shun me or turn me away because I haven't been the best follower over the years?

*While praying one day, a woman*
*asked, "Who are you God?"*
*He replied, "I am love, I am grace, I am*
*peace, I am joy, I am strength."*
*"Now I understand, but who am I?" God tenderly wiped*
*away her tears and whispered, "You are mine."*

*—Author Unknown*

I have always believed in God, except for that one semester in college when we were studying world civilizations. Our professor had some lively conversations in class about the Mesopotamians and Iraq, the *cradle of civilization*. Like a typical student in a liberal arts course, I soaked it all up like a sponge. I think most college professors are agnostics or atheists as well as *uber* liberals.

They shape the young minds of their students who then go out into the world with their inflated liberal spirit, nonstop zeal, and a burning desire to provide for all the downtrodden. Someone told me once that no one becomes a conservative until they are responsible adults who understand how the global economy works. Until then, money is a commodity that is to be given away to any cause.

## Why Is Mesopotamia Called the Cradle of Civilzation?

 Mesopotamia is generally credited with being the first place where civilized societies truly began to take shape. Situated in a vast expanse of delta between the Tigris and the Euphrates Rivers, Mesopotamia was the wellspring from which modern societies emerged. Its people learned to tame the dry land and draw sustenance from it.

—Josh Clark, www.howstuffworks.com/history 2014

Trying to be a sophisticated college senior who had an open mind and not much experience in critical thinking, I accepted his lectures *in toto*. Never did I question any of this. I fully believed that out of this delta came a wellspring of belief in Gods and religion was born.

These Gods were a necessity to rationalize all the unknown events of great magnitude, like floods, famine, pestilence, wars, etc. These forces of nature were cruelly powerful and the Mesopotamians had no control over them. It's somewhat logical they would assign all these adversities to powers beyond themselves, their omnipotent *Gods*.

It was such great rationalization! Thus, they had a God of lightning, a God of war, drought, famine, etc. I tended to regale my noncollegiate friends of all these facts as though I was suddenly an expert on ancient civilization. Far from it. I never thought, for one minute, *where did these superstitious Mesopotamians come from?*

Had I thought of that, I would likely have to admit that a greater spiritual being was involved in the creation of man and earth. Man, being given free choice and free will, decided to create various Gods to explain events beyond their comprehension at that time in history. They prayed to these Gods to help control their environment and sustain their existence.

And so, organized religion as we know it began to take shape and form. I believe that today's organization of churches continue to exist on the large scale they've evolved into, as much to meet man's earthly needs as to serve God. One only has to consider the vast amount of wealth amassed by these entities to see that. Church heads are treated as demigods, many of whom live in splendor. Jesus didn't live in splendor or have gold spun robes. They don't seem to be patterned after Jesus. It seems, instead to be an affectation that may have arisen from egos that became bigger than the Gods to whom they pray.

# Ode to Angelo and Mary

My parents Angelo and Mary,
A couple quite contrary!

Married early in their teens,
She was barely seventeen!

Three children by the age of twenty,
They had so little, yet they had plenty.

Angelo's good looks and zest for life,
Made women jealous of his wife.

Angelo worked long hours in the coal mine,
Mary had three babies and a full clothesline.

He left the mines after a deadly mining disaster,
Hearing the rush of water in his ears, he ran faster.

He swore he'd never again go down that dark hole,
Too many men were entombed in that crush of coal.

Mary took a sewing job when she was fairly young,
Working in a factory where vicious gossip stung.

Seasoned workers saw her as naïve and easy prey,
She worried she wouldn't have the fortitude to stay.

Her earnings were meager, his got slightly better.
She never quite fit in, he was a "go-getter."

Artistic, nurturing and gentle in her way,
The two of them were like night and day.

He was strong and healthy, never sick a day,
She had many an illness come her way.

There was one thing they both did quite well,
Graceful when dancing, they held all in their spell.

Mary's confidence withered as her frailties grew,
Childlike and defenseless, she was often blue.

Angelo didn't comprehend nor fully understand,
Withdrawing emotionally, off to others he ran.

Mary never said a bad word about anyone,
Angelo was cynical and full of prankish fun.

Angelo was the backbone of this union,
He blamed her when their plans fell to ruin.

They saved a little bundle to build a new house,
He was excited to plan for his kids and spouse.

But savings were used up for hospital bills,
Mary needed surgery, doctor's care and pills.

Disappointed, Angelo grew quite bitter,
He felt his life had become a "no-hitter".

Toiling years in the coal mine seams,
He felt robbed of all his dreams.

Mary was often the target of his wrath,
She'd unwittingly set him on a warpath.

Daunted by mounting medical bills,
Mary felt overcome by all her ills.

One day it became too much,
She longed for a loving touch.

Though she loved her family very deeply,
She took many pills and got way too sleepy.

Mary recovered by a wing and a prayer,
People she knew would whisper and stare.

Mary was just content to stay at home,
As he aged, Angelo had no desire to roam.

On retirement, he took over the heavy chores,
Learning to write checks, he shopped the stores.

Mary seemed happiest with her family around,
A debt-free Angelo held his head high in town.

Life was less stressful now toward the end,
He became Mary's cook, caregiver, and friend.

The day came this once strong man lay dying,
Deathly pallor cloaked him where he was lying.

Despite his lost and oft-troubled wife,
He saw in her the true love of his life.

He reached out weakly for Mary's hand,
She smiled weakly, too ill to understand.

In the very end, when any hope was grim,
He needed her more than she needed him.

I have had a stop-start, intermittent relationship with the church since my childhood days. I had the great misfortune to have a few conflicts with our parish priest who was incredibly frightening to me as a young girl. He totally scared the bejesus out of me with every single encounter! He had slicked back hair and rimless eye glasses which he used to burn a hole in you as he looked at you in disdain.

He seemed to enjoy having that kind of power over helpless, naïve children. Despite that, it never shook my faith in God, just the church. I knew that God was a supreme being who loved all of us. I'm not at all sure we were loved by this priest. He seemed hostile toward us and brimming with sarcasm. I guess God had his reasons why he allowed this particular priest to preach to us, but I can't think of one.

So in the days of the Mesopotamians, they revered their Gods who were perfect beings, not flawed like man. Their Gods had the power to save man or annihilate him. By their own creation, they sustained their faith through a mix of fear and reverence and through a belief in the supernatural. I prefer to think of God as loving and gentle, but with almighty strength that would never be used against man, only to support him, guide him, and reveal the way and the light through this labyrinth we call life.

*I am the way and the truth and the life.*
—Jesus to his Apostles at the Last Supper; John 14:6.

In the '60s, God was fear; in the '80s, God was love. What a dichotomy the church created! It's no surprise that my participation in the mass wavered during those earlier schizophrenic years of *hate vs love*. The vast organization of churches and dioceses was suffering from some sort of identity crisis during those decades. Well, maybe not all churches, but certainly those of the Roman Catholic faith.

The mass was done in the Latin language which no one but the altar boys and the most diligent of Latin scholars understood. But it was beautiful and had a lyrical quality to it that I loved—*anno domini, et spiritu tuo, in excelius Deo . . . Kyrie, Kyrie . . . I could still hear it and smell the incense!* The priest said the mass and we followed. We were happy to be their flock.

Fast forward to the '80s and the large-scale changes that did away with the Latin mass, converted everything into English, and whisked the parishioner onto the center stage and into the heart of the mass. Laypeople now assist with the offering of Communion and the Chalice of Wine—the body and blood of Christ.

This is quite a privilege for someone not wearing a cassock and priestly robes! The Gospel and reading of scripture were turned over to lay members of the parish as well. The priest only had to show up on Sundays and Holy Days to deliver his homily, the sometimes painfully long sermon following the reading of the scripture.

The sermon is usually tied to a lesson in morality for those attending mass to take home and chew on. I find that some of them easily become guilt trips; after all, who among us has not sinned or faltered? The priest is bound to hit a nerve with fifty-two or more sermons to deliver each year.

Sometimes, I wonder if he looks around the room as he delivers his homily to see if anyone's head is bent especially low, avoiding eye contact. Then he might think to himself, "There's one, a man with the burden of guilt so heavy on his shoulders they sag. He needs to get into the confessional soon."

Prior to this new era of enlightenment in the church, the members of the parish were totally under the heavy hand of the priest. I remember in the early '60s everyone at mass was asked to stand up, raise their right hand, and repeat after the priest a solemn oath not to see the movie *Peyton Place*. It was popular at the time and thought to be scandalous in its content. As teens, we were all trying to get our hands on the book, as we doubted we'd ever get in to see the movie. Compared to today's novels, it was pretty tame.

There was some dialogue that involved mention of a young girl's breasts. This was something that was taboo in this pre-hippie, bra-burning era. Once the war protestors broke out and began demonstrating about free love, the antithesis of the violence of war; I just wonder how many would keep or even take that kind of oath. I don't know how many broke their solemn oath after mass that Sunday, but I would venture a guess that more people wanted to see it *after* the oath than *before*.

In today's society, there are many deities, multiple religions, and corresponding churches with their recognizable architectural styles, and as many belief systems as there are ethnicities. Every culture has a religion. These stained glass structures, temples, chapels, and other places of worship are adorned with many iconic, earthly symbols of adoration and heavenly creatures. There are statues of saints, crucifixes, chalices, candles, menorahs, baptismal fonts, choirs with organs, confessionals, etc.

We really can't do enough to honor those we adore. I wonder sometimes if it has evolved beyond reason. I don't know the answer but feel overwhelmed by the history of competition between various religions and sects. There is still a mind-set of *my religion is better than yours*, or *my God is better than your God*. And some deities are quite antagonistic toward one another. This has been the impetus for wars and rebellions throughout time.

When I think of the pillaging, hangings, torture, imprisonments, large-scale bloody battles and devastation of entire villages and surrounding environs, I cringe. So much violence in the name of religion! It reinforces my tendency to feel put off by the *institution of the church,* some of which have teachings that are entirely oppressive. So when I say I turned to God, I didn't look for him to be waiting for me in the pew of my local church.

Currently, I do belong to a church in my community. I like to go there to focus on and communicate with God in a more reverent way than I can at home. I still like some of the trappings of the church, especially the stained glass windows. When the sun is shining through them, I almost feel like a miracle can occur and God might show up and walk right through that window on a beam of sunlight.

The environment is suitable for prayer, soul-searching, and meditation. I like praying there and often tell God, "Please God, I need you to hear my prayers and help me. I know you can't take my cancer away, just help me to be strong toward the end." Although, I have to admit, there are moments when the priest sounds too preachy and self-absorbed. If he's also delivering a too-long-to-absorb sermon, parishioners will begin squirming in their pews and some will bow out early or avoid him like the plague.

Whether I continue there or not, I'm praying that when I pass from this earthly world, my guardian angels will lift me and carry me to heaven where I can reside with God. I just hope he hears my prayer. I may not deserve it, but I'll be indebted if I could live forever at his side. Faith in God will help me face death openly and with dignity and to go peacefully from this earthly realm.

That prayer and the vision of my angels comfort me and sustain my strength to continue on this journey to its predictable end. I believe in a spiritual afterlife. In fact, I recently read a book about a woman who died, went to heaven, but came back to her earthly life because she was told her purpose had not yet been served. It's a very vivid account of what heaven is like and how the angels interact with humans to help them here on earth. I find this quite fascinating!

Others have written about these near-death encounters and describe what that light is all about at the end of the tunnel. There are such similarities in all their stories that I choose to believe them. They make sense of life as we know it, the implications of death, and a spiritual afterlife. One such account was written by a spiritual woman who was an orthopedic surgeon and mom to four children. This is a highly educated person who clearly was in the presence of God and then sent back to fulfill her mission on earth.

There are good and evil forces in our lives and most of us have the human need to believe in something more powerful and wonderful than we could ever imagine. It lifts us up. These wonderful celestial beings, all invisible to us, represent the Heavenly Father here on earth. They help to protect and guide us throughout our earthly life. They are waiting in the wings when our lives come to an end. Then they move in, ever so gently, to transport our souls toward the light to a heavenly place where we can live among God and the angels. This is what I believe and it's what I will hold in my heart as I take my last breath.

*Let us endeavor so to live
that when we come to die,
even the undertaker will be sorry.*

—Mark Twain, American Writer

# The Mass B.C.

As a child, I always did what I was told,
If I attended mass on Sunday I was gold!
In those days we followed the Golden Rule,
We didn't have thoughts then of being "cool".

But nuns and priests were so awfully strict,
Not at all like the liberal ones they now depict.
We had to walk a very straight and narrow line,
Or get kicked out, which was a shameful fine.

Women wore lovely hats to show respect for God,
No one at the time gave it a thought or felt it odd.
Shouldn't respect be about what you "said" or "did"?
Well, heck, what do I know, I was just a kid!

If you forgot your hat, it was like you were naked and exposed,
You had to borrow a hanky and keep your mouth firmly closed.
You must never draw attention to yourself or talk during the mass,
If you do, you're sure to be humiliated in the next catechism class.

Don't even think of whispering while you're kneeling in the pew,
The priest will rap your knuckles with the bible and hiss at you!
It seems to me everything we did was committing a mortal sin,
With any infraction of the rules, they'd call our parents in.

One summer day while I was kneeling at the Communion rail,
The sacred host fell down my summer dress as I caught holy hell!
A stern warning was "spit out" at me to see the priest after mass,
This incident left me embarrassed in front of my catechism class.

It wasn't a faux pas on my part, I think it was more his error,
But I agonized over it during mass, a sheer hour of terror.
Two silent nuns retrieved the errant wafer on a golden plate,
My dress dangled at my waist as I shivered, dreading my fate.

It was quite an embarrassing scene for a budding girl,
Not yet wearing a brassiere, it made my head whirl!
The priest later smirked at me, but silently let me go,
Running home, my pounding heart was beating so!

There was another incident two years later after school,
Entering the church, I blessed myself in the vestibule.
As I moved forward, I was yanked back by my scarf,
It was the same scary priest, I wanted to barf!

His hair slicked back, his eyes so piercing and cold,
I thought he looked like Satan, a fearful sight to behold!
He said loudly that I blessed myself using my left hand,
He claimed it was a sinister act, but I didn't understand.

It was a totally unconscious action on my part,
I'm just a left-handed child, not an evil dark heart!
He wanted to know if I was praying to the Devil,
How can he say such a thing? Is he on the level?

Once again, I was completely humiliated in front of my class,
Why couldn't he just turn the other cheek and give me a pass?
The third and final incident was to be my biggest sin,
While waiting for the weekly catechism classes to begin.

Word spread quickly which priest was on his way to the church,
It was Satan's clone, not the docile one; it made my heart lurch!
Many of us split and took off just like "desperados" on the run,
By morning, calls to parents of each "truant" child had begun.

It seems we were roundly kicked out and would all go to hell!
Those weren't his exact words, but he meant that just as well.
He demanded a parent to bring us to the rectory to apologize.
I went reluctantly; I could not look this icy man in the eyes.

I muttered my fervent lament with my head bowed low.
I'm sure he thought this penitence was all part of the show.
He knew I'd show remorse, I was cornered like a scared rabbit!
I longed to escape from this tyrannical man in the black habit.

All these events occurred long before my diagnosis of cancer,
But it's why I drifted from the church looking for more answers.
I could no longer belong to a church that bred fear and hellfire,
I was seeking the love of God in a place that would inspire.

After cancer, I attend mass because it now comforts me,
I pray not for myself but for all my friends and family.
As for me, my terminal illness is a foregone conclusion,
Of that cold hard fact, I entertain no delusions.

I pray for souls, whose lives are not yet decided,
They may need help if they become misguided.
I also pray for those who departed before me,
May their souls be at peace and their spirits free.

There is symmetry to the mass that appeals to me,
It flows just like tidal water going back out to sea.
The priest, a man of God, dressed in robes unfurled,
Preaches love for one another and peace to the world.

How different it is now as though someone waved a wand,
To remove former harsh penances and warnings so strong.
Being at mass now, I need not be just a casual observer,
I feel welcome to participate as a reader or a server.

The priest's blessings fall like warm summer rain,
It lifts my spirit and allows my soul to soar again!
How divine it is to find my faith is still so strong,
In this place where I feel safe and that I belong.

Now I can celebrate the mass without any fear,
I have no one to taunt me or make my eyes tear.
I can sing hymns or pray with total abandon here,
In this House of God that I now hold so dear.

*The Angels were all singing out of tune, And hoarse
with having little else to do, Excepting to wind up the
sun and moon Or curb a runaway young star or two.*

*—Lord Byron*

# SECTION 9

# MENTAL CHANGES

Mental changes presented mostly in the form of *chemo brain,* the unavoidable fogginess, forgetfulness, and memory loss that plagues many people after several rounds of chemotherapy. I don't know if these toxic drugs singed some of the nerve endings in my brain or gray matter, but I simply cannot remember some things I never had a problem with before. Some people who have this syndrome have to use Post-it notes on their car's dashboard to remind them how to get to work, even if they've been driving that route for years without difficulty. I have lists for everyday reminders.

Often, I forget the names of people and places, what I did two minutes ago, details about where I've been recently, remembering my purse or sunglasses as I leave restaurants of just about anywhere that I set it down, what movie or TV show I watched yesterday, or leaving my cell phone, glasses, or jacket in a variety of places. My husband fills me in a lot with dates, names, and details. He also gives me reminders and goes back to look for my purse or phone or glasses. What would I do without him?

There are the mental changes brought about by stress. Initially I experienced a bit of anxiety about what will happen next, the inevitable fear of dying borne out of a growing apprehension for the eventual separation from my family, my loved ones, my close friends, and my loyal and dedicated dog Flora. She has stuck to me like glue since this all began. The part that hurts the most is that I know I won't see my grandchildren grow up. What will they be like as young adults? What careers or employment will they seek? Will they marry and have children of their own? Will they move away or stay close to their family roots? Will they be happy and lead productive lives?

> *Cancer changes people. It sculpts us into someone who understands more deeply, hurts more often, appreciates more quickly, cries more easily, hopes more desperately, loves more openly, and lives more passionately.*
>
> *- Author Unknown*

Other changes in my life after cancer that resulted in stress are due in part to the experiences I had with certain tests and diagnostic procedures that were uncomfortable enough that I dreaded ever having them repeated. I hope that I don't ever have another breast MRI. It's one thing to be stuck in a huge metal tube for an MRI for over an hour. It's quite another to be on your knees inside a giant metal circular machine with your head facing down and your arms extended out in front of you, like a submissive, sacrificial lamb in a sadomasochistic ritual.

I was at least *fifty shades of pink* before it was over! Both of your breasts are hanging by gravity into two separate clear plastic compartments for visualization purposes during the MRI.

The feeling of vulnerability is beyond belief—who designs these machines? Are they typically women-haters? Misogynists on a mission? Masochistic narcissists?

And if that isn't bad enough, your face is resting on a plastic padded doughnut that makes you sweat, just in case the sadistic equipment and posturing itself isn't enough to get those sweat glands working overtime! About thirty minutes into the test, I had a trickle of sweat rolling ever so slowly down my cheek. It made me feel itchy and I wanted to swat it like a fly!

I was warned not to move, even the slightest, or they would have to repeat the test. It felt to me as though several lifetimes passed by before that trickle stopped. By then, I was sweating bullets, so it was immaterial. I was just one big puddle of flop sweat and would prefer death by hanging than to continue with this torture. Not to mention that my arthritic shoulders and knees were none too happy with this grueling challenge.

The last source of stress, but likely most important, is the worry about my husband. We have been through this together and he has become my caregiver and has been very supportive of me. He has remarked in the past that he'd be lost without me. That thought doesn't make me feel at all good.

I dread thinking he might go through his days without purpose or direction. I have pretty much been the "fire starter" at home. I plan our trips and vacations and most often select where we should travel or what destinations we should see. I take care of our banking, bills, and budget. He often defers to me on major decisions. I don't want him to be alone and hope he finds someone to fulfill the remaining days of his life.

Planning for this eventuality included setting up files that I hope he can use to find important papers and information when the need arises. I know that he has no interest in learning about it now, but this should help him later on. I think he has always wanted to make me happy, so he went along with many of my wishes. We make all decisions together, but he'll often say, "Do whatever you want," or "Whatever you think is best."

I've seen what it does to him if I'm gone for a few days. He sort of roams around the house, doesn't eat as well as he should, doesn't sleep well or sleeps too much, most likely on the couch with the TV on to keep him company. In general, he loses interest in doing any of the things we might have done together if I was at home. My heart truly aches that I'll have to leave him some day. He has made me the center of his life, especially since my diagnosis. Maybe our daughters will come through and involve him in their lives.

He cooks for me, shops wisely to make sure I'm eating a good, anti-cancer diet, cleans, and does a lot of the chores I used to do, like watering the plants. I'm hoping that Flora will fill his days with companionship and love. She is very attached to me but has made a lot of progress with him since we adopted her over seven years ago.

She was approximately two years old at the time, according to the best estimate of the *Waggin' Tails Sanctuary*'s dog-rescue staff. She was very afraid of males. My husband, Gene, couldn't approach her without her barking and growling incessantly at him till he backed away. To his credit, he was very patient. It took almost four years for her to make any sort of breakthrough with him.

Now, she gives him lots of kisses (licks) and will follow him each morning, panting and tail wagging, to get her morning treats. He'll always say, "What's Daddy got for his little girl?" She just loves it, and it seems to be mutual. Bedtime has become her special time with him as he gives her brisk tummy rubs that she just loves! He feeds her in the evening and provides her with fresh ice water three times a day. They've come a long way.

We think she may be part *diva* because she won't drink stale or warm water. She likes her *water on the rocks*! She loves that refreshing taste of cool water with a few ice cubes floating around in it! We can laugh at these idiosyncrasies now. But we weren't amused when we first adopted her.

We were appalled that she had been abandoned and likely abused. She had been living in the streets, begging for food several days according to accounts from the dog sanctuary. She was probably drinking rain water from puddles. We feel she deserves to be spoiled. We get so much unconditional love in return from her.

Flora

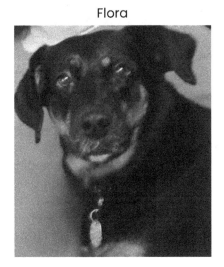

Flora seems to have an obsessive-compulsive disorder as well as a post-traumatic stress disorder from whatever abuses she endured. We assume she was abandoned, but she may have run away from a home where there was no loving care in store for her. She was very frightened of running water and would run and hide whenever I turned the shower on.

Banging of pots and pans or sudden loud noises unnerve her. Loud screaming or shouts reduce her to shaking from head to toe. She will run to a safe place or *hidey hole* if she is exposed to angry words. We don't yell at her and don't hurt her in any way. But I get the distinct feeling that her former owner had done quite a bit of that.

She has these little rituals that must be done in a precise order. When I give her a special treat, she won't eat it unless I'm sitting right there with her. If I'm gone for the day, she will keep it close but will not touch it until I'm home. Then, when I settle into a chair, she'll eat her treat, but not until she puts her paws on my knees and licks my face first. I think it's her way of saying *thanks*. Also, I have to stay with her to watch her eat the treat or she'll stop right in the middle of it. Then we have to go back to step one where she jumps up to put her paws on my knees and licks me again.

Once, I had some phone calls that interrupted this ritual more than once. We had to repeat this exercise four or five times from the beginning each time until she ate her treats. If she has a treat left over from the day before, she'll line up her treats in a neat row and always eat the older one first. She has a great sense of orderliness for a dog. She also has a fairly large vocabulary and always seems to know what we're saying to her.

She seems to saying *Mom* sometimes when she is anxious for attention. At least it sounds that way to me. Like many dogs, she also is good in knowing what we're thinking about before we say anything and will react in kind. She'll run and hide the moment we start thinking about giving her a bath or brush her. I suppose many house pets are like that. She also knows when we're going out long before we leave and will sit in a corner very quietly until we go.

After we leave, she jumps up on our bed and digs into the bed clothing to build a little fort to hide inside. I guess it makes her feel safe. Usually she runs out to greet us, but one time she must have been in a deep sleep. I walked quietly into the bedroom. When I called her name, her head popped up from behind the bank of covers she had gathered. It was actually kind of cute and comical. She looked surprised and relieved at the same time!

Another interesting behavior we observed in Flora is how she reacts to the removal of her dog collar. She has metal tags on her collar that make a jingling sound whenever she walks or scratches herself. My husband jokingly calls it her *neck jewelry*. Occasionally, we have to remove it to replace the rabies tag with a new one or to bathe her. She is visibly upset and acts like a she has just lost her last friend.

We think it might be that she is worried we'll give her back or abandon her like the previous owner. When we pick up the collar and put it back on her, Flora becomes very animated. It links her to us and us to her. She prances around and then, suddenly full of energy, bounds through the house like it's Christmas morning. I think it's pure *doggie happiness*. She is clearly delighted to have her *jewelry* and collar back on.

Recently, I told my husband that it's a lot like *Wonder Woman* of the comic book fame, who becomes infused with super energy and special powers when she puts on her tiara and gold wrist bracelets. From the time I was a young child, I was fascinated with *Wonder Woman*. Who wouldn't be? She had a knockout body, pretty face framed by curly hair, an invisible plane, a golden lariat that made criminals tell the truth, a golden eagle spread across her ample chest, and knee-high red boots that are to die for! She can run like the wind, toss that lariat, and round up a whole posse of crooks in a flash, then fling her tiara at some evil thug and nearly decapitate him.

My first connection with this female icon of strength and veracity was a second hand DC comic book a relative gave me from a stack his daughter used to read. I read it over and over, becoming submerged in this Amazonian woman and her legend more each time. I wanted to be her. I grew up and somehow put aside that preoccupation to complete my education and make a *big girl* move from Pennsylvania to New York. Despite my trepidation, I accepted a really appealing, but challenging administrative nursing job in a large medical center located an hour north of New York City, in Westchester County.

At the time, I felt like I was in water over my head and might not do well managing the demands of the job. I wasn't concerned about the clinical aspects of the role. It was all the non-nursing *procurement* responsibilities that worried me. My predecessor had set up the job in a rather odd way. Much of her time was spent ordering supplies from various vendors. It could be anything from heart valves to pigskin for burn cases to tubing for suction or disposable garments and drapes for staff wear or patient use in the Operating Room (OR).

This was foreign to me! It was a county government system of procurement with bids and a dual-tracking system. It involved a set of numbers when the bid was submitted and a purchase order number when the bid was accepted. It took a long time to obtain items as all this paperwork had to go through a maze of red tape before it could be filed away. I became that clerical person and knew it had to change soon. I did not go through all those years of nursing education and clinical experience to be tied to a desk as a super mega clerk and procurement agent for the OR!

That's when *Wonder Woman* (WW) resurfaced in my life. In hindsight, it may have been a subconscious desire to gain super strength by emulating my idol. Or it may have just been coincidence when I bought a *Wonder Woman* nightshirt. But it was no coincidence when I received a *Wonder Woman* book in 1974 from friends on my thirtieth birthday. I think my two buddies sensed I needed a little bucking up! The introduction was written by Gloria Steinem. It was published by Warner Books as a *Ms Book*. Pretty iconic! Right? Wow, that entire woman's movement seems totally ancient now! But the subconscious message to me was that I needed to be strong in this new role.

It took patience and the right timing to convince my administrators that I was better suited and much better utilized overseeing staff and doing the assessments, planning, and implementation of hospital and nursing policy in this administrative role. We were able to hire a clerical person to do my former portion of non-nursing responsibilities. Sue became a great asset and freed me up to assume the other pressing challenges of my role.

I also had the able assistance of JoAnn whose role included troubleshooting the logistic problems related to booking surgical procedures. Her ever-expanding clerical duties were a great aid to me. It was good timing as all the administrative nursing roles were soon to change. I subsequently became the assistant director of nursing for the recovery room and the intensive care unit, in addition to the OR. The only thing that is certain in life is change.

In time, I got a 2001 printing of another book about *The Golden Age of Wonder Woman*. These books both contained reprints of older comic strips. Personally, I prefer the vintage look to the current modern, sexy-looking woman with sensuous curves and leg-baring blue tights. I've received some pretty good swag from close friends and family over the years. I now have a fairly representative, although not extensive, collection of WW paraphernalia.

It includes a rather impressive WW action figure with golden lasso, a thermal mug, a huge red ceramic cereal bowl with the WW logo on it, a wooden hand-painted trinket box, a full-length apron, T-shirts, wall art, pop-up books, miniature invisible plane, magnets, and metal pins.

On my most recent birthday, my seventieth, I received a new book about *The Secret History of Wonder Woman*. The book explores twentieth-century feminism and was written by a *Harvard* historian and *New Yorker* writer, Jill Lepore. She claims *Wonder Woman* is the missing link in the history of the struggle for women's rights. Pretty serious stuff and it all began in 1941 with a comic book!

They say you prioritize your life differently after you've had a terminal diagnosis. I'd say that's inevitable and certainly out of necessity. You no longer have that open-ended feeling that you'll be around forever. There's an expiration date that's been slapped on your chest so you are keenly aware that the clock is ticking. You want to do more with your life before the clock runs out on you. Not knowing exactly when that will happen makes this the cruelest game of all. There's nothing like having the *Grim Reaper* at your heels to give you a sense of foreboding.

Every time I think of booking a cruise or planning a vacation that's months into the future, I know it's a gamble. By the time it rolls around, I could be sick due to a recurrence, or worse, I could be ready for *end of life care* because my medications and their alternatives aren't working any longer. A woman with mets said that 2015 was going to be a good year for her. She passed away three weeks later as the New Year started. *Carpe diem!* Seize the day and make it yours! When my cancer becomes resistant to all the available drugs for my estrogen-sensitive tumors, it will signal the need to call in the services of hospice. I think about it now for a *nanosecond*. Then I go ahead, make the plans, and book the cruise. I'll take my chances and kick cancer to the curb!

Currently, I have plans that blanket the entire year and don't feel any anxiety that I won't make it. You can't live your life in fear of all the possibilities, and no, I'm not going to be prompted to say to you, "Tomorrow I can get hit by a bus or a car and die." Well, now I've gone and said it, but I don't mean it. It's the most frequent phrase people like to throw out at someone who is newly diagnosed with metastatic cancer. I can't help but feel it's an offensive comment. The probability of that happening to them is one in one million. The probability of my dying from cancer is one in one—big difference, *don't you think*?

*Life is not always a matter of holding good cards, but sometimes, playing a poor hand well.*

—Jack London, American writer

# Report from the Front

The situation on the frontlines
Is looking pretty grim,
Sisters and brothers are falling,
And survival is looking slim.

Battered and tattered from
The onslaught of warfare,
They are subdued and praying,
In their foxholes of despair.

I've been on the frontlines,
Of this millennial-long war,
Spent hours in chemo trenches,
Almost forgot what I'm here for.

Had numerous rounds of ammo,
Enough to kill every live cancer cell.
At times I felt I'd rather give up,
Than endure this tortuous hell.

Next we're going nuclear,
Gonna bomb this thing to hell.
Cause when I make my mind up,
I truly want to get well!

Not all of us win this battle,
Some are on the front many years.
They have to change strategy often,
As the enemy force has no fears.

The enemy is a chameleon,
It changes its toxic mix to fool us.
We have to be brilliant,
They continually school us.

Just what will it take,
To annihilate this terror?
Who will lead the charge?
And become the standard bearer?

*CAROL A. MIELE*

What's the secret weapon,
To defuse this enemy's power?
Will it take a gargantuan bomb,
Nuclear fission or radioactive shower?

They've used toxins,
Chemicals in every vein,
They steal your sleep,
And cause you more pain.

Maybe an act of God
Needs to stop this war.
A pure ray of light from above,
Signaling it's worth fighting for.

I think I'll hold out,
For the next wave of recruits,
Hopefully they bring with them,
Bigger guns and better boots.

We just need more time,
And a better offensive plan,
Then we'll totally obliterate,
This heartless killer of man!

*Because I could not stop for Death,*
*He kindly stopped for me;*
*The carriage held but just ourselves*
*And immortality.*

—Emily Dickinson, American Poet

## SECTION 10

# EMOTIONAL CHANGES

'm quite familiar with the diagnosis post-traumatic stress disorder, or PTSD. It became a frequent diagnosis in the post-Vietnam era. At one time in my nursing career, I worked in the psychiatric unit of a veterans administration hospital where military men, mostly Green Berets, and military women were treated for this disorder. It was a difficult condition for them to live with and for everyone around them to get used to.

For starters, their behavior was marked by a *hair-trigger temper*, and under certain circumstances, they would start swinging in an explosive fit. You don't want to be the nurse who has to awaken this soldier from a sound sleep. I would call to these patients from the doorway rather than the bedside until I got a response. It worked well for all involved. It was a good thing, as I was pregnant at the time. Most of them were quite polite and even protective of me if, by chance, a delusional, psychotic patient got too close to me or acted in a threatening way around me. The problems they exhibited mainly occurred during sleeping hours due to horrific nightmares or upon awakening.

Now, there is a new term from experts called *post-traumatic growth* or PTG. It's pretty much the opposite scenario, as this is used to describe people who have struggled with a major life crisis, like cancer, and whose life changes for the better. They develop a new perspective and actually become stronger in terms of those things I discussed earlier: psychological, spiritual, and emotional changes. Those who experience PTG may even dedicate the remainder of their life to a cause. Or they may pursue those things in life they truly wanted to do that eluded them in the past.

They hone their coping skills and zero in on that which makes them happy. I feel I can relate to this and see how my spiritual side has especially begun to evolve into a search for my personal angels here on earth. I actually think they have sent me messages in the recent past. Like the St. Christopher's medal I found lying on the floor of the back seat of our car.

We rarely ever have back seat passengers, and those who were said they have never seen this medal when asked. Neither one of us owned it or had ever seen it. But there it was, giving us a prayer for our safety on the road. I feel it's so special. Another example is the way I am aggressively pursuing painting, drawing, writing, and poetry. I know that I wasn't as driven before as I am now. I feel more determined to accomplish those things I avoided or put off before. Tick, tick, tick.

Do you know if you possess *resilience?* Do you know what this word conveys? It's defined as the ability to recover quickly after a setback or when something really bad happens to you. *Resilience* is a great thing to develop while dealing with a cancer diagnosis. This is a quality I wish for every person experiencing cancer to possess. It's a hard road to travel without it.

Along with that, it helps to have strong core beliefs, a strong sense of and a belief in self, as well as faith and a deep and reverent belief in a higher power. For the body to fully heal and recover, consider the obvious mind-body connection many people disregard. The mind and body come in one package and they do affect each other immensely. So if your body is trying to heal, but mentally you're not accepting your illness, you may not heal as quickly or as well, if at all.

I observed this concept firsthand when I was growing up. Whenever we lost an important football game or basketball game when I was in high school, I saw a lot of sad faces on the field or on the court, and I often wondered how the players could suit up again, face their opponents and the fans, and play their best game.

There is an old Chinese proverb: *Mistakes pave the path for improvement*. So without fail, at the next game, they were standing tall and played as well if not better. I don't know if it was the locker room pep talks or something else. I believe what I saw was a resilient group of kids who had learned to roll with the punches and learned a lesson or two along the way to improve their game.

It's hard to roll with the punches when you're sick and in treatment for cancer, but that's what you must do. Sobbing every time I thought of my grandchildren or the words *bone metastasis*, I recognized I was in a dark place and didn't want to stay there. I did eventually go on an antidepressant. It was suggested to me by someone who was diagnosed nine years earlier with the very same mets I had. I wasn't suffering from major depression, but I needed a lift out of that dark hole and away from my sorry state of mind.

Once I started on it, I was able to handle things so much better and to feel that I was more in control. Just being able to stop the flow of tears frees you to do things, including extensive research about your illness. Knowledge is power. I intended to gain as much power as needed to accept and understand what was in store for me.

I like to think that I have developed a positive mental attitude about living with cancer. Although, I still feel somewhat jaded about the medical industry's lean record of cures with cancer treatment. Just keeping it real! Once I felt emotionally stable, I became more vested in pursuing things I love to do, like painting and writing. Doing these things makes me happy. It takes all the raw emotion and drama going on in my head and translates it on paper. It's a great outpouring for me and it seems to also help others who read or view my work.

But not all of us have the capacity to become stronger after something tragic like cancer occurs. The inability to rise above it can negatively affect the outcome of treatment. I look at it this way— what is the other option? Lie down and die? I believe that if the will is broken, the body will follow. You can take that to the bank.

My will is very strong and I don't give up easily. It's just not in me to cave in. I have too much living to do. I also have a lot of catching up to do when it comes to traveling and seeing places I haven't seen before. I would enjoy that simple pleasure of seeing glorious sunrises and sunsets in various parts of the world.

If you don't have it in you, connect with people that do. You'd be surprised at how it much rubs off. When I went for my first chemo treatment, I was still a broken woman and couldn't believe I needed to actually go into a cancer center for treatment. In my line of work as a professional nurse, I was accustomed to providing treatment to cancer patients. It felt odd now that I was to be on the receiving end.

The first patient I had a conversation with at the cancer center was in a cubicle right across from me. The nurse had just asked me my birthdate as part of the safety checks before giving me medication and starting the chemo infusion. When answering the nurse, my new neighbor's head perked up. She heard me say my birthday was on Christmas day, hence the name *Carol*. It turns out she was born on Christmas Eve and was named *Christina*.

We had a bond now. She turned out to be the best medicine for me. She was spunky and brave with a great attitude. We chatted during most of my treatment time and it just flew by! When I think about her now, I don't think it was a coincidence that we met. I think it was divine intervention. Thank you, my guardian angel.

Christina told me she was forty-one years old and had three small children. She was young, by my standards. I felt pretty bad about that. At least my daughters were young adults and independent. She said she would soon be getting a "tummy tuck and a boob lift". At first, I didn't get it. Then she explained they were excising and pulling up a full thickness of skin on her abdomen to create a flap (graft) for reconstruction of her breast.

The breasts were going to be "perky" according to her. And she would have a smaller, tighter abdomen as an added bonus of the procedure. She was going out the next evening to celebrate her last chemo treatment. She said, "I drink and smoke when I go out. I pretty much do whatever I want. Life is too short."

Part of me shuddered when she said this, but another part of me admired her moxie and free

*CAROL A. MIELE*

spirit. We chatted again as she was leaving, I could feel all the energy in the room leave with her. She advised me before our *good-byes* not to think about my cancer when I left the center and went home. She added that I should make a habit of not thinking about it at all it in between appointments and just live my life.

As she waved at the door, she called out, "Carol, put cancer on the end of your shoe and kick it to the curb!" It's probably the best piece of advice I've been given since diagnosis. I took that lesson home and embedded it deep it into my psyche. It would become the driving force of my recovery from the grueling days of chemotherapy and into the more comforting phase of remission.

> *From one man, he made all the nations . . .*
> *So that they would seek him and perhaps*
> *Reach out for and find him.*

—Acts 17:26–27

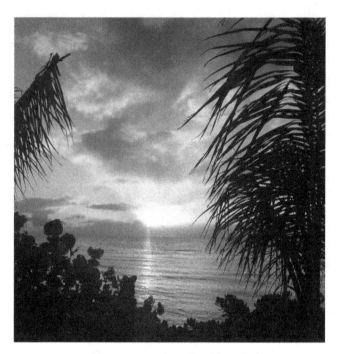

## THE CANCER COLONY

The Cancer Colony is a picturesque, idyllic island in the Pacific Ocean. Privately owned, it boasts spectacular sunsets and year-round ideal weather. A very desirable, attractive, and relaxing place for anyone to inhabit, especially people with metastatic cancer, but there is one problem: this place and this story is wholly fabricated by me. I hope it may come to pass someday.

The idea for this *Utopia* occurred to me when I was communicating online with several women who have metastatic breast cancer (MBC). These women were lamenting about the callousness and total insensitivity of certain people they know well. These people either avoid them ever since they learned of the cancer diagnosis, or they say things that are very hurtful regarding their illness. They complain that some people don't believe them because they "don't look sick enough."

I have made contact with many women with MBC through various web sites that are set up as virtual support groups. I go there almost daily for the unique opportunity to share what we have in common due to our illness: problems, fears, family or financial issues, and treatment side effects. We also share our joy when there is something to celebrate, like a new scan that shows the cancer is stable and there is no new cell growth. The camaraderie we share is invaluable.

Sites like this help in so many ways, from the peer support of people walking in your shoes, to more in-depth support from cancer advocates or experts on cancer care, who so often are a part of the supporting network on these sites. When indicated, they serve to assist in clearing up confusion bringing information to the group, like a new clinical trial or a recently approved drug on the market.

Perhaps there's a side effect you're having a problem with and someone in this group may have had experience in resolving it. The support and the feeling of *we're all in this together* goes a long way toward helping our *metsisters* and *metsbrothers* adapt and adjust to their new reality.

There's nothing like advice from someone who knows intimately what you're experiencing. There is unconditional trust in such groups and the bonds can be pretty strong. Some of these groups are *closed* or *private*. Members need to know they are *safe* to say what they're thinking. Often, it's a close family member or friend they need to vent about.

It could be very damaging to have that person mistakenly, or purposely, enter this site and read what's being said. Also, when a member passes on, it's good to know that the solitude and commemoration of that person's life isn't interrupted by a nonmember with a funny story to tell. We respect each other and know enough to temper what we say with the right tone at the right time.

As a result of this level of confidentiality, there is great comfort with disclosure of sensitive issues. So the issue of disregard some people show for the person going through this ordeal was recently discussed widely. Often, I read a post from someone having a bad day who notes that it's good to feel you're *not alone* in this, or how terrific it is to have people to share your fears or concerns, or to be part of a group of people who totally "get it."

There have been a number of people, both men and women with MBC, that I've had communication with. They have expressed openly the vast lack of understanding by others of their metastatic illness. We don't expect them to know all we know and have learned, but they could take an interest and learn something, as we did.

Metsters are invariably exposed to insensitive and stinging remarks from close acquaintances. On one level, there is realization that the comments were not meant to be painful. But on another level, the pain of hearing it said by someone you thought should know better is devastating. These caustic remarks may or may not break down the friendship but will cause a great deal of grief and turmoil in the life of the injured party afterward. The words will be repeated over and over in their head for days.

The worst part of this scenario is that cancer patients need to avoid stress in their life. Cancer is impacted by the immune system and vice versa. It can become too easily compromised by stress. When you're already dealing with a terminal illness, it can exacerbate things just as the person is enjoying a period of remission. It may not activate the cancer per se, but many of the side effects can be exacerbated. It puts a strain on your whole being when you least need it.

Who knows what causes the cancer to come back? We don't know why we got it in the first place! One woman said she went home and cried all evening after a harsh comment by an acquaintance she ran into who said, "You're still here? I can't believe that you're still alive!" Some avoid going out in public places to avoid these well-meaning friends.

Others have expressed, euphemistically, a desire to live in a place where the only inhabitants are people *like us* who understand, don't judge, and would never say the *wrong* thing. Join me now in this fictional *Shangri-la* where *metssisters* and *metsbrothers* from everywhere and anywhere can congregate, cohabitate, and comingle in peace and harmony. I know I'm a bit if a dreamer, but without dreaming, we lose the excitement of possibilities!

*Yes, I am a dreamer. For a dreamer is one who can only find his way by moonlight, and his punishment is that he sees the dawn before the rest of the world.*

—Oscar Wilde, Irish Poet and Writer

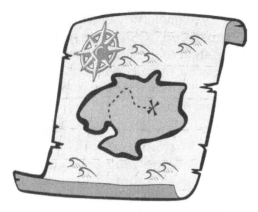

## LIFE IN THE CANCER COLONY

The Cancer Colony inhabitants will have very little need to worry, feel frightened, or have anxiety. This select population will have, at their disposal, every day if needed, specialists and professionals to take care of any and all problems. No insurance preapprovals or managed care negotiations to deal with. There are no deductibles or co-pays. No long commute to obtain treatment as there is a *Cancer Chute* system that delivers the patient to the door of the specialist or healthcare professional via a people transporter system.

This system is connected throughout the island with easy access from bungalows and villas, at reasonable intervals. It offers safe, comfortable rides in plush *Care Cars* on a high-speed rail system or *Chutes* that deliver you right to your stop! Anything that can potentially happen to you is controlled for, anticipated, and safely managed by a dedicated staff of nurses, oncologists, social workers, psychologists, pharmacists, dentists, chaplains, nutritionists, clerical staff, and technicians.

An undertaking of this magnitude essentially involves great visionaries who have vast holdings, numerous resources, and tremendous dedication to come together for the sole purpose of creating the *Cancer Colony*. They're motivated to assure that cancer patients will be treated kindly and holistically. Funds from donors, moneyed people with very deep pockets, and humanitarians provide the capital for this venture. Most are on board because they lost someone they loved to cancer and want to make a difference, while honoring their loved one.

This would be a truly remarkable and monumental accomplishment. Meeting all the complex needs of people with advanced cancer is challenging. These needs are psychological, physical, spiritual, emotional, financial, and social in nature. Just the task of gathering together a diverse group of people that have this one undeniable thing in common, terminal cancer, is a phenomenal undertaking. But to do it well and make a positive difference in the quality of these lives, you must admit, is incredible! That's my vision.

Let me clarify something first. This wouldn't be some sort of *penal colony* or a *leper colony*. Inhabitants who volunteer to live on this island wouldn't be treated like recluses. Nor would they be treated like undesirables, such as the dredges of society no one wants living next door to them. They would choose to be there, to have their needs met in a nonjudgmental, open-minded, and unbiased way.

It means freedom—freedom from the stigma of having terminal cancer and the predictable "sad eyes" that follow you in your home or wherever you may go. And it would mean freedom from the speculation about how long you have to live, how many more months, weeks, or days you have left, how many birthdays, Christmases, or anniversaries you might yet have to enjoy, how your family will manage without you, and how long it will be before your husband or wife remarries or your children forget you.

These and many other questions are not just written on the faces of the people you know or meet, but they are often spoken, in hushed tones, or in random conversations, as though you can't hear them. Like, "I don't think she really has cancer, she never lost her hair," or "She doesn't look sick enough to have cancer."

Cancer doesn't cause deafness, stupidity, or insulation from getting hurt. It doesn't make you nobler, smarter, saintlier, braver, more honest, or stronger. Cancer just makes you very sick. Then you die. Well, eventually you die.

Despite all the awareness of breast cancer, the phenomenon each fall known as *Pinktober*, has not overcome the dearth of misinformation out there. This is a national campaign involving those ubiquitous pink ribbons that adorn just about everything, everywhere during the entire month of October. It's an enormous campaign, yet there still exists a general lack of clarity regarding the types of breast cancer, the risks of cancer, what metastasis is, or that it's incurable, what the symptoms are, etc.

There is almost no knowledge in the general population that metastatic means it's incurable and, therefore, terminal. Most people don't know that a breast cancer spread to the lungs is not actually lung cancer, but breast cancer that has invaded or metastasized to the lungs. There is a corresponding lack of knowledge about how breast cancer can present itself. My first symptom was itchiness of the breast. Until then, I had no knowledge it could be a warning sign.

Most people don't really want to hear how serious your illness is or that it's not possible to *beat it*. And if you don't, it's not your personal failure. It's beyond your control! They don't want to be faced with their own mortality or to be reminded that it could be *them* next. They can't help it.

People tend to keep their cards close to their chest. We're also in the era of HIPAA, the Healthcare Information Portability and Accountability Act that allows steep penalties for divulging anyone's private health information. And it's human nature to be protective. So it's become the cultural norm. Therefore, I have to ask, "Why can't we change the norm?"

Many other cultures handle death and illness with much more openness. They see death as a normal part of the life cycle. It's a natural and expected ending to our existence as we know it. It certainly should not be something buried deep in the psyche or whispered about like some taboo topic but spoken of with thoughtfulness and compassion.

It should be allowed in open discussions—not in closets or back rooms, but in the nest of family togetherness. In our society, we value privacy to an almost obsessive degree. And we keep things hidden, sometimes with the notion that we must be strong and shield others from our pain. These are people I call *martyrs*. I don't think we need people to martyr themselves when the important topic of certain death is on the table.

I don't believe this notion serves anyone well. People who are uninformed can't be expected to respond appropriately to a person in a dying situation. We've prevented them from doing so. Also, for the patient, often thought of as the *victim*, they aren't getting the level of support or understanding they need. We have prevented that by not informing them in the first place. It's their right to know.

Unless we're looking for bravery medals, this *Code of Silence* interferes with any chance of facing and coping with a very personal tragedy. No one should have to martyr themselves to spare others. Everyone should be on the same page, at least to the extent that they have the capacity to understand and absorb the information.

Families function better when they are all included in important matters that affect them. This is particularly true when crucial decisions are being made during a family discussion. It's an upheaval in the family dynamics. The shockwaves will be felt by everyone. So everyone must be prepared and proceed accordingly.

Secrets can be toxic and could do a lot of damage. I recall a time, at least three decades ago, when the norm was not to tell the person who had cancer about their diagnosis, or heaven forbid, that they were dying. The rationale was it would worsen their quality of life. They would give up. They would get worse. They would die sooner. Or perhaps they would become morose. We would never forgive ourselves for telling them. These and other outcries have been used to justify keeping the diagnosis sealed.

Then there is the person who doesn't want to know. This is the person who is in denial and too frightened to hear the truth. I recall when I was in a situation like this with my own father. He was dying of extensive Stage 4, inoperable gastric cancer. He didn't seem to be picking up on the clues we were giving him or asking any leading questions about his illness. My sister Dee and I met with him one day at his primary physician's office to tell him about his grave diagnosis and the poor prognosis.

We wanted to explore it further with him if he showed any inclination that he wanted to know. Our feeling was that we needed to help him plan for this eventual outcome and involve him to whatever extent he chose. At the time, my mom was in a nursing home following a month-long hospitalization and narrow escape from death. She had emergency surgery, became septic, and was unconscious and on a ventilator in the intensive care unit for a week.

It was clear that our parents were in crisis. That's troubling enough, but to have these life-threatening illnesses occur simultaneously was heartbreaking. Our brother Sam lives in Georgia and could not be there to deal with this face-to-face confrontation. We explained to my dad that he had a large tumor in his stomach that was inoperable. We added that there was no treatment for it, other than management of his symptoms, and that this was due to the extensive nature of the tumor.

He sat there like a deer caught in the headlights. He stared straight ahead, not making eye contact with any of us. I could tell by his wide- eyed expression that he was frightened of what we might say next. He was not a great communicator, and in this circumstance, he was like a sphinx and withdrew from the discussion. He neither wanted to talk nor wanted to hear anyone else talk. He wanted a quick escape route back to the safety of his house and familiar environs! We were at an impasse.

I remember that same wide-eyed, naïve look he wore every time one of his siblings died. He had outlived several, in fact, all but one of seven sisters and brothers. They all died of cancer. He looked very pale and became completely quiet. After we disclosed that he had a large tumor that had been growing in his stomach for some time, we asked him what questions he had. This was the perfect opportunity for him to let us know he was ready to hear whether or not he had cancer and/or was dying.

He shook his head *no* and looked straight at the door leading out of the office. He could not wait to get out of there. He was not going to be a willing participant in this tragic scenario, even though he was the central character.

We left feeling we had failed but couldn't force this very grave information on him if he wasn't ready to hear it. A week or so later, he called my oldest daughter Marisa to ask her. He always seemed to be able to talk more openly with my two daughters than with any of us.

He wasn't quite as reserved with them as he didn't feel he had to be the strong father figure. So he was more playful and carefree with them. With prodding, he was even able to tell them "I love you." This is something he was never able to tell me or my two siblings our entire lives, although we knew he did love us.

He was from that tough, but silent generation of men who bit the silver bullet, even when in severe pain, before ever giving in to it or yelling out in anguish. Finally, a week or so later, he called my daughter Marisa, to ask her if he was "a goner." She had to tell him he was. I felt bad that it fell to her, but he was ready then and clearly preferred to hear this news from his granddaughter. Timing is everything.

My belief is that we must find a way to prepare people so they can make plans to get their lives in order. There are pre-payment funeral plans that could be put into effect that would lessen the financial burden for the survivors. Decisions can be made about the funeral arrangements and the burial, if so desired.

Some people have preferences about how they will be dressed or what should be placed with them for their *final sleep*, such as a favorite pair of rosaries or prayer book, photos of children or grandchildren, a locket from a loved one, etc. They can update their *Last Will and Testament* and put an *Advance Directive* or healthcare proxy in place.

They can get all of their affairs organized while they are still mentally and physically capable of doing so. None of this can be accomplished if we keep the truth hidden to *protect* our loved ones from their own destiny. They may not have a lawyer, life insurance, a burial plot, or an undertaker. They need time to make preparations and may need support; but the final decision should be theirs.

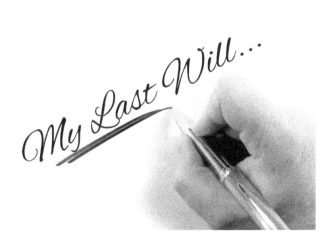

# Living in the Cancer Colony

Joining a group of people on a remote island,
Who all had my illness did at first seem odd.
But soon I came to understand that all of us,
Were to become the special "Children of God.*

Basking on a sun-drenched beach,
Bathed in sunblock, or lolling in the water.
We find the weather is always perfect,
It needn't be either colder or hotter.

Fresh foods growing on the island,
Meet all our nutritional needs.
Fresh fruits, vegetables, fish and fowl,
Just picked nuts, sprouts and seeds.

We have found a Paradise for the transition,
From our earthly life when it is our time.
There's no sadness here as we're joyful,
We'll all get to make that heavenly climb.

All our symptoms are managed,
By a crack oncology/palliative care team.
They combine herbs with traditional medicine,
And have treatments with a proton beam.

There is zero tolerance for pain here,
It's the Cancer Colony's Golden Rule,
Using patches, drips, pumps and pills,
Or gentle waterfall therapy in the pool.

Massages with palm oil or acupuncture,
Reiki applied by grand masters of the art.
Visual imagery, meditation and Tai Chi,
Soothing Zen-like music fills the heart.

Sleep is never a problem when we recline,
We're on the finest of air flotation beds.
And slumber in balmy warm breezes,
As ocean waves lulls our sleepy heads.

To fulfill our spiritual needs, Angels Chapel,
Keeps its doors open both day and night.
Our Guardian Angels watch over our souls,
Their trusting countenance never out of sight!

There is no "Pinktober" here, nor a sea of pink,
No pink products, ribbons, walks or races.
No more dreading an entire month,
Filled with celebrations and happy faces.

We're all on the same page here,
We have no fear of awkward greetings.
Whenever two or three of us are together,
It's like a spontaneous support meeting.

Living Wills and Last Testaments,
Are drawn up by an army of lawyers.
They're done online, as are estate sales,
And will readings promise no "spoilers"!

Visitors are always welcome here,
They arrive daily by cruise ship or plane.
The Cancer Colony knows their importance,
These contacts effectively eliminate any strain.

We have memorial burials on floral floats,
They go out to sea just as the sun sets.
Anyone can take part in scattering the ashes,
Go aboard and take along favorite pets.

Religious rites and requested ceremonies,
Are always followed and respected.
Our multicultural community,
Gets along peacefully, as expected.

Some say it's a magic potion in the water,
Or that it's the rare purity of the air.
Whatever it is, the Cancer Colony,
Offers compassion beyond compare.

We accept that, until our purpose is served,
This life's a mere stop along the way.
True joy awaits us at God's side,
Beyond the swirly Milky Way.

We live an enriched life here,
Still we long for that glorious day.
We'll slip beyond the tendons of Angels,
And wing to our spiritual hideaway.

Once we arrive there,
Cancer's damage will be gone.
We'll rejoin others that came before us,
And we'll all sing their heavenly song.

The Cancer Colony is the perfect Utopia,
Yet it exists only in my mind.
Though I yearn for it to be the place
Where these souls are enshrined.

*Born in the fire of the counterculture movement of the '60s,
the reference Children of God was a spiritual revolution fueled
by an all-out commitment to God. They developed a unique alternative
society that was uncompromising and unconventional.*

—www.childrenofgod.com

# SECTION 11

# THE WAITING GAME

L ife is a rather long waiting game—we wait to be born, wait for the first cry, and wait for numerous *firsts* the next twelve months: first smile, laugh, word, steps, foods, liquids from a cup, etc. As we get into the school years, it's the first day of school, the first best friend or play date, first sleepover, first boyfriend or girlfriend, first formal date, first dance or prom. I could go on about life's *firsts,* but cancer pumps up the intensity of the waiting. You wait for the results of biopsies, MRIs, scans, lab results, etc. The worst is the sense you are waiting to die.

You no longer have any life goals now other than staving off death for as long as possible via medications and/or treatments. Time is not on your side. It marches on, ticking away the minutes that you will no longer have. You think to yourself, "They told me three to five years. I'm getting to the other upper end of that range. Might next year be my last?" I've heard of a number of deaths from MBC recently. Many of them seemed such vibrant people, so alive that they defied all the projections, yet they indeed succumbed a relatively short time later. The clock had run out for them—tick, tick, tick, tock.

But I decry, I have so much to do yet! I have not reached the pinnacle of my life. I'm not ready for my emotional nadir. I must be spared so I can continue on this path to self-realization, to bring good deeds and words to mankind. I must have more time to leave my mark upon this earth. Yet I realize these entreaties are my singular effort to negotiate the terms of my living and dying—*Morte e Vida*. I have already reached the third stage in dying as described by Elisabeth Kübler-Ross in her 1969 book *On Death and Dying*.

She outlines five stages of normal grief. In our bereavement, we spend different lengths of time working through each step and express each stage with different levels of intensity. The five stages do not necessarily occur in any specific order. People move back and forth between these stages before achieving a peaceful acceptance of death.

The first two stages are *denial and anger*. I experienced that early on and did a darn good job of it—just ask my family! I even told my oncologist that the analysis of the first PET scan was all wrong—these weren't cancer cells in my left scapula, head of the right femur, thoracic, and lumbosacral spine, pelvis, ribs, and sternum. This is all a big mistake! This supersensitive test is not perfect by any means, I thought.

The PET scan must have picked up inflammation in those areas and read them as cancer cell growth, tumors. I thought it could be inflammation because I'd had falls and various injuries in the past involving these locations. Some resulted in bursitis or tendonitis. My body has old war scars there, not cancer, I rationalized.

My oncologist quietly took all this in and gave me the benefit of the doubt. She ordered an MRI of my thoracic, lumbar, and sacral spine along with an MRI of the pelvis. I felt a sense of relief that she not only believed me, but also thought this could be plausible. *Way to go, Carol! You've already got cancer on the run!* Except that I didn't.

The report came back clearly identifying scarred osseous tissue in all these areas that are typical of damage left behind by cancer cells that have feasted on your bones. It's similar to the pock marks you have left on your face or body from a bout of chicken pox in childhood. The story goes that if you scratch them, you will be scarred for life—at least that's what most moms threaten their children with when they insist on scratching away.

The third stage is *bargaining.* It's a fairly normal reaction to the feelings of helplessness and vulnerability you feel at this point in your life. It's justified. After all, isn't your very life being threatened? You are about to go down that slippery slope. You are frantic to regain control and put on the brakes or come to a screeching halt. You may even be inclined to make a deal with God in an attempt to postpone what is becoming clearly inevitable.

Your mind is filled with *if only* thoughts. If only I had gotten that mammogram earlier. I did put it off for a few months due to a more pressing need for medical attention. If only I hadn't gained that extra weight right after I retired. It serves me right! I was enjoying my free time too much and eating snacks any time I felt like it. I silently said at the time, *God will get you for this.*

Now those words have come back to haunt me. The snacking frenzy fueled by the freedom I felt after retirement wore off after the first month or two and likely had no role in my developing cancer. I've learned that weight gain can be a risk factor for postmenopausal breast cancer. Some estrogen is produced by the body's fat stores. The more estrogen a woman has circulating though her body after menopause, the more she is at risk for breast cancer. I do wish I had known that.

It's likely, however, that my cancer started long before that. This negotiation stage is actually a feeble attempt to protect oneself from the painful reality that is beginning to settle in.

For the curious, the fourth and fifth stages are depression and acceptance. I've got those covered as well. An antidepressant worked wonders to lift my mood and to stabilize it so I didn't cry every time someone asked about my diagnosis. It was quite helpful to me as I began the transition to a stage whereby you simply make peace with it. I didn't say you become friends with it and want to hang out together—just that you finally accept it so you can move on to the more important aspects of your treatment and just taking care of yourself.

As soon as you've done that, go out and have some fun! Book that cruise. Go on that vacation, take up a new hobby, get out and make new friends, don't just stop to smell the flowers, get out and plant some, put them in a vase when they've grown so you can not only see them, but smell their beauty. You'll benefit from the fresh air, the vitamin D, and the great feeling that comes from working with the soil and giving the promise of life to some beautiful flowers and plants. Your guardian angels will love you for it and perhaps God will be smiling down on you as well.

*There are four corners to my bed,*
*There are four angels overhead.*
*One to watch, one to pray,*
*Two to lead my soul away.*

—Author unknown

# Flight 2014: Wings of Hope

In 2014 I fumed, "Cancer researchers
are still in pursuit of the Holy Grail!"
Every year I hope this will be the one
That science succeeds; every year it fails.

Time flies by while new drugs for longevity,
Slowly and almost painfully creep along.
These drugs in the pipeline add just days,
To our lives, so I must stay strong.

Many do their level best to support me,
But they are unable to understand.
It ravages you, breaks your spirit and,
In the end, forces your hand.

Only you know how it feels,
You'd sell your soul to be well again.
"Stay positive," they say glibly,
Oh, how much these words offend!

They urge, "Don't lose hope!"
It just makes me think,
Why hang on to hope?
It's a thread not a rope.

To challenge this belief,
I set out on a quest.
Took a leap of faith,
Gave *Wings of Hope* a test!

Began this journey somewhat naïve,
Not prepared for twists and turns,
Or steep climbs and sudden plunges,
That made my stomach churn.

We dove into the Depths of Despair,
Gliding across misty Waterfall of Tears.
We passed solemnly over the Valley of Death
Through the dark and murky Veil of Fears.

Wings of Hope followed rippling currents,
Over the swelling waters of Chemo Creek.
We veered off as the chemically infused,
Toxic smell made the sweet air reek.

Onto Radiation Ravine which proved,
To be the scariest terrain of all.
Clinging tightly and white knuckled,
I prayed I wouldn't fall.

Atop the surgically sculpted Slippery Slope,
We endured moguls and a meandering ride.
Lumpectomy Lift to Mastectomy Mountain,
By going across the Great Sternal Divide.

Onward, we navigated through a maze,
Of "Pay As You Go" pharmacy aisles.
Pills, capsules, syringes and vials,
Crammed on teetering shelves for miles.

I was overwhelmed as I saw long lines,
At the Cancer Center and Oncology Labs.
But no less depressed by the rows,
Of lifeless bodies on mortuary slabs.

At journey's end, I felt hopeless,
And running out of time.
Had more questions than answers,
Now isn't that sublime?

Cancer was lurking long before,
Hieroglyphics were drawn on cave walls.
No cure despite the billions spent,
Is a harsh reality that truly appalls!

Metastatic Cancer is terminal,
There is no turning back.
I pray for a miracle breakthrough,
Before my world turns black.

*CAROL A. MIELE*

I also pray for the "mets" sisters,
And brothers standing in my shoes.
We have our prayers and candles,
But so very much to lose.

Post-Flight Questions

Why must so many suffer with Cancer?
Will someone please give me an answer?
Is the cancer industry simply too big to fall?
Would a cure bring financial ruin to them all?

Would stocks tumble and the Dow take a dive?
Should every cancer patient suddenly survive?
I say this not serendipitously or facetiously.
My questions could not be posed more seriously.

*Oh sovereign angel,*
*Wide winged stranger,*
*Above a forgetful earth,*
*Care for me, care for me.*

—Edna St. Vincent Millay

# FLIGHT PLAN FOR FLIGHT 2014: WINGS OF HOPE

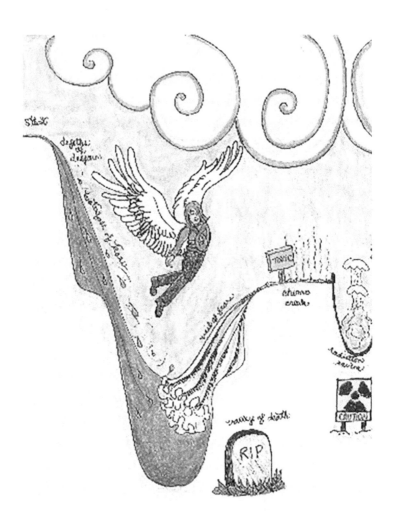

*CAROL A. MIELE*

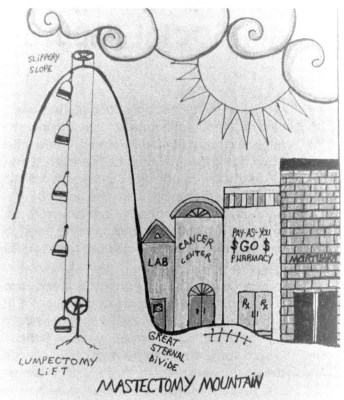

SLIPPERY SLOPE

LUMPECTOMY LIFT

LAB

CANCER CENTER

PAY-AS-YOU $GO$ PHARMACY

MORTUARY

$R_x$   $R_x$

GREAT STERNAL DIVIDE

MASTECTOMY MOUNTAIN

FLIGHT ON WINGS OF HOPE

## SECTION 12
# RANDOM THOUGHTS AND SOCIAL MEDIA

This book is an eclectic collection of memories, innermost thoughts, future visions, constructive criticism, dreams, and wistfulness. There is no central, overriding theme or moral. There is just one principle character: its name is *Cancer*. I'm not the voice of my generation, but I am the voice of one with metastatic breast cancer. I am driven to do what I can to shine a light on the pressing need to study the cascade of events that cause cancer cells to metastasize.

When we learn that, meaningful steps can be taken to stop the metastasis and prevent it in those with early stage cancer that was *successfully* treated. People don't die from early stage cancer. They die from Stage 4, advanced, metastatic cancer. And of those who were cured from early stage breast cancer, 30 percent will go on to metastasize. Nearly 40,000 men and women die each year of metastatic breast cancer.

Despite the billions of dollars that have been raised, that number has not changed appreciably in the last three decades or so. The need goes from pressing to desperate when one realizes that many of these are young moms with babies. Their cancer is more aggressive. They have not even had the luxury of screening and its *game over* for them.

This is a reality at a time when one should be able to expect more from science, medicine, and its combined wisdom.

Helping us to live a few more days or weeks longer is no longer an acceptable resolution. That small, incremental gain just extends the suffering while waiting to die. What we need is to stop cancer in its tracks, not just slow it down! My social media contacts are proving to be sadder and sadder, which makes me feel angry. So many young women dealing with Stage 4 breast cancer are dying. It's so discouraging to hear nearly daily about another death of a *metsister*.

One person I have come to know through social media, Linda Lou Batchelor Ballew, was kind enough to put together a *Scared e-mail* to help those who are newly diagnosed. She posts it now and then to help buoy sagging spirits and inspire them to feel there is some hope amid the grim details. So much of our healing and ability to go on is connected to how well we cope with this diagnosis.

Linda was born in Hastings, England, but came to the United States to live with her husband, Peter. They have two daughters who still reside in England and a son who lives near them in Indianapolis, Indiana. At sixty-seven years of age, she has seen a lot and has carried her own share of burden. She once worked actively as a registered nurse, but a back injury and Stage 4 cancer restricted her to life in a wheelchair these days. I laud her for recently receiving her American citizenship! Here is Linda's letter.

# The "Scared" e-Mail

For those who are new, scared, or just having a tough time and feeling scared right now:

I went regularly for eighteen years, twice a year, for my checkups. I felt I didn't belong. I was an impostor with the women there suffering with what had long left me. Then July 9, 2008, my markers were up. No one seemed bothered, so I began running around getting tests done. All negative. After five months of rising markers, the oncologist did a CT/PET scan: five nodes were positive in and around my lungs. "Is it cancer?" I asked. He told me he was 80 percent sure it was.

Then my world collapsed. I didn't want lung cancer. As a nurse, I had cared for many who had lung cancer—not that for me! I had a whole life and people to care for. I remember the anger, fear, numbness, tears in the middle of the night, gripping and heart stopping despair. Then they found the severe bone marrow mets and gave me a three to four month prognosis. Suddenly the lungs were the least of my troubles. Nine months later, still alive with no treatment, I had ten to twelve months to live.

To call me scared was a gross understatement. Then I met others who were Stage IV and they were living. They were just going for treatment and living. They too had felt as I had, and yet day by day, life moved on. Planes didn't fall out of the sky, cars didn't run off the road, the sun rose in the east and set in the west. I realized I could live at least day to day. They were living proof.

You have come to the right place and a local support group will help if you have one. We can manage this; it is another stage of our lives, like childbearing and menopause. Every day a treatment bubbling on the cauldron of trials and FDA approval appears on the market and for some or another of us it brings more time, even NED (No Evidence of Disease), a stable time when nothing changes much and our body is normal again. This is not the end. It is the beginning of a journey with sisters and brothers who tread a different path than they did before, with a deeper love of life and tiny everyday activities.

We have all been in the early days of shock. Gather your information. Come and talk to us about it. Many on this site will be on the same treatment. We cry with you and hold you in our hearts until the first days grow longer and time brings you to another place. Tell us where you are, what doctor you see. We are all over the world. Maybe someone shares your doctor or treatment or lives where you do.

I send you prayers of comfort for the night time, and blessings of new life visions for the day time. This happened to us because we are human—no crime was committed. Nothing you did brought this on. Stop searching your mind for the unanswerable— you are among us now and we will help you. Keep posting and tell us what is happening, how you are doing. We will be waiting to hear from you.

Much Love and Gentle Hugs,
Linda BB, Indiana

*She'll come at dusky first of day . . . And I will follow her away.*

—Francis Ledwidge, Scottish Poet

## Author's Note of Acknowledgement

I am so grateful to Linda for sharing this supportive letter for newly diagnosed people with metastatic breast cancer. It has just the right tone for the very frightening early period that one goes through when it's all new. There are so many scary thoughts that pop into your head.

Your mind is racing and you constantly ask yourself why this happened? Is it from something you did or something you didn't do? You can make yourself crazy if you don't establish some good lines of communication with others.

Chatting online with people who are going through the same thing is very beneficial. We all help and comfort one another.

# METASTATIC MEANDERINGS

The Mission

- I have *possession* of all my faculties when I say an act of *commission* is not the same as an act of *omission*: one is a willful act, one is a failure to act.

- The *conclusion* is that treating one for Stage 4 cancer so they can *transition* to *remission* is job number one.

- To refuse or decline treatment or to not receive it for any reason is an *evasion* of one's rights. This is not to be confused with *submission* of a DNR (Do Not Resuscitate) document which addresses emergency situations while one is hospitalized.

- To treat someone with cancer, one must have *permission*. The *emission* of toxic drugs into the bloodstream cannot be taken lightly. It would be a serious *transgression* to do so without consent.

- There must be signed *permission* of the person who needs the drugs. The physician's order then becomes a legal *transmission* in the patient record. Only then can the *submission* of the patient for the chemotherapy take place.

- It may not require an *admission* to the hospital as it's largely an outpatient procedure. On occasion, there is an *intermission* to give the patient a break from this arduous regimen. The *mission* or goal is to put the patient into *remission* from their cancer, at least for a while.

- Hearing you have advanced cancer can cause an *implosion* in your life. *Explosion* wouldn't be the right word because everything suddenly comes down on you—the dust and smoke doesn't clear up for weeks, or months.

- I don't wish to cast *aspersions*, but this cancer gig sucks! An apt *assertion* is that it seems we're light years away from a cure while I have just a few left.

- Many cancer patients suffer from *depression*. Some will withdraw into *seclusion* at home. Others make the *decision* to ask their physician for an antidepressant. If open to the *suggestion*, there are help lines that are open twenty-four hours a day, seven days a week, if they choose to call for support.

- My *confession* is that I did all of the above. The first two months after diagnosis, I didn't go into complete *seclusion*, but only mixed with family. While on chemo, losing hair, energy and some friends, I wasn't feeling very sociable. The right *medication* boosted my spirits, and when I no longer needed the antidepressant function, it worked magic with hot flashes one gets from Aromatase Inhibitors.

- Oncology is an admirable and honorable *profession*. You may not always see your patients get better: many will die. But you will have helped them through the most difficult time in their life. That's a heady and weighty thing when you think about it.

- I think you have to have a *passion* for what you do to do it well. That combined with *compassion* for their patients makes for the perfect oncologist. At least it does for the ones who've treated me.

- I don't have the *delusion* that I'll escape this disease or the illusion that I'll die by other means. Stage 4 is pretty black

- and white. But on *occasion* I think maybe I'll be among the one percent who actually gets better. I don't have an *obsession* about this thought, just a pleasant *sensation* when I do think about it.

- I once painted a *procession* of women with their IV poles in hand, following God down a path. The *assumption* is that they aren't alone in carrying this burden, that God was with them, sharing their burden. I hope it's a comforting message.

- It's been my *impression* that Stage 4 patients do so much better when they are given love and support. The *erosion* of the family unit in this country has left many without this emotionally based advantage. They are suffering much more than they should be as there's no one to provide *distraction* or *diversion.*

- My *compulsion* is to reach out to everyone going through this, to touch their hands and reassure them it will be all right. But it won't really be all right. As cancer goes through a process called *progression,* in which the cancer continues to grow after it has become resistant to the medication, nothing on this good earth can hold it back.

- It will consume healthy tissue until you can no longer sustain major functions. There may be *obstruction* of systems or *occlusion* of vessels, even *compression* of bowels or effusions of lungs can occur. No blood *transfusions* or antibiotic *infusions* will change that. The die has been cast. This sounds awful, but it's truthful. We all need to prepare for the eventuality of our demise. Say your prayers, make peace with someone, check that your *pension,* savings, or investments are safe and intact. Use this *occasion* to put important documents together, and take time for *reflection*. Be at peace with yourself.

# Ten Things Not to Say to Someone With Metastatic Breast Cancer

1. Gee, you look great! You don't look like you're supposed to be dying.

2. You're still around? I'm really surprised! I thought you'd be gone by now.

3. You're going to beat this! Those doctors don't know you. They just say all that stuff to cover themselves, just in case.

4. I know you have cancer, but you would not believe the awful week I've had!

5. Not for nothing, but whattaya gonna do with those wigs? I mean later on. I could really use them.

6. Do you think your husband (or wife, girlfriend, boyfriend) will marry again? How soon do you think he'll (she'll) wait?

7. So have you found out yet why you got cancer? Is it from smoking when you were a teenager?

8. So what's up? It's been four years. I thought they told you two to three? Does this mean you're cured?

9. I could help you by taking all those clothes you that can't wear anymore off your hands.

10. Your poor kids (husband)! God bless them. (him) How will they (he) ever get along without you?

# Ten Things to Say to Someone With Metastatic Breast Cancer

1. Let me help you out by shopping for your groceries this week.

2. I want to help out while you're in treatment. How about a hot casserole? I can bring it to your house every Wednesday night.

3. I can take you to the cancer center and stay with you for your next treatment.

4. Need any books to read? I have a lot at home I can bring over to help you rest better in bed and to make sure you don't overdo it.

5. Call me whenever you have prescriptions to be picked up. It's no problem for me to drop them off at your house for you.

6. I've arranged to add your name to our prayer group for our weekly prayer meeting. We're all pulling for you.

7. I'm doing laundry tomorrow and thought I'd take yours home with me. I can return them tomorrow, folded and sorted.

8. Why don't I come by one day this week to do some light housekeeping? I can dust, mop, and vacuum. What day is best?

9. I can take your kids to the zoo Saturday or a matinee on Sunday. It will give you some quiet time with your husband and an opportunity to rest. Let me know which they would prefer.

10. I can't possibly know how you're feeling going through all of this, but I'm a good listener. Tell me how it's been going for you.

# Twenty Things that Make Me Cringe

1. People who are mean or abusive to other people.
2. People who are mean and abusive to animals.
3. Dishonest or greedy people.
4. Mold, mildew, or rust.
5. Liver, in any shape or form!
6. Bad hair or makeup days.
7. Cliques, snobs, or haters.
8. Nail polish smears and spills.
9. Getting oily stains on clothing.
10. Clothes that make me look frumpy, old, or fat.
11. People who don't flush the toilet after using it.
12. Traveling at night in fog, rain, or icy conditions.
13. Shoes that are too tight or squeak when I walk.
14. Bossy or pushy people who won't take "no" for an answer.
15. Spilling coffee on my clothes while driving to an appointment.
16. Sushi, calamari, or anything squiggly that comes from the sea.
17. Drivers who rush out in front of me, then slow down once there.
18. People and food workers who don't wash their hands after using the toilet.
19. Stains on the front of my clothes that can't be covered with a scarf.
20. Callers who don't identify themselves, thinking you should know who they are.

# Thirty Things that Make Me Smile

1. Gentle summer rain.
2. Golden autumn days.
3. Crickets on starry summer nights.
4. Sounds of a refreshing waterfall.
5. Dipping my toes into a babbling brook.
6. Crossword puzzles and word games.
7. Chicken pot pie or homemade soup on cold, wintry days.
8. Pizza, pizza, pizza anytime!
9. The sound of ocean waves.
10. Reading indoors on a rainy day.
11. Photos of my grandkids.
12. Birds in flight formation going south for the winter.
13. Sounds of chirping, whistling birds in the trees.
14. The sweet smell of a newborn baby.
15. The feel of a baby's soft, smooth skin.
16. Wizened faces lined with character.
17. Flowers in my garden or spilling over my windowsill and trailing in planters.
18. The aroma of fresh-baked apple pie.
19. Snuggling with my dog Flora.
20. Nuzzling with my husband and getting gentle kisses on my neck.
21. Balmy breezes on warm days or at night.

22. Clothing that makes me look leaner or sharply dressed.

23. Shoes that make me look taller.

24. Good hair and makeup days.

25. Smell of fresh coffee grounds.

26. Fresh snowfall that glistens in the sun and looks like a soft blanket.

27. An ice storm at sunrise turning everything into a crystal sculpture.

28. Soft, billowy clouds as seen when lying on my back in the grass.

29. The scent of fresh pine while walking through a wooded area.

30. The feel of the surf running through my toes as I walk in the sand.

# Carol's Song

Aromatase inhibitors keep the cancer away,
A bar of dark chocolate really makes my day.

A sluggish port flush makes me feel uneasy,
And when it's blocked, I can get quite queasy.

Subcutaneous injections strengthen my bones,
Anti-inflammatory painkillers deflect the moans.

Fresh fruit and veggies, high protein, no sugar or soy,
The anti-cancer diet still leaves a lot left that I enjoy!

C'mon, Cancer, I defy you to break me down,
C'mon, Cancer, I'm so ready for a shakedown!

# SECTION 14

# HOW THE NUMBERS STACK UP

- Prevalence—The number of people living with metastatic breast cancer in the US is estimated to be 155,000–162,000, but no statistics are currently collected.

  *Prevalence is the number of people living at a given point in time who ever had a breast cancer diagnosis.*

- New cases—The number of new cases each year of metastatic breast cancer is unknown but consists of those initially diagnosed Stage 4 and those who had early stage breast cancer and have a metastatic recurrence. Approximately 6–10 percent of new breast cancer cases are initially Stage 4 or metastatic. This is sometimes called *de novo* metastatic disease, meaning from the beginning. Men represent approximately 1 percent of the new cases.

- About 62,570 new cases of carcinoma in situ (CIS) will be diagnosed annually; CIS is noninvasive and is the earliest form of breast cancer.

- Mortality—About 40,000 will die from breast cancer. They will be Stage 4 at death. There has been no significant decrease in the deaths in the past few decades. With 813 women diagnosed daily, 110 die every day.

- There is one death every thirteen minutes in the US from breast cancer. (Komen website)— All deaths from breast cancer result from the spread of breast cancer cells to other vital organs such as bones, lung, liver, or brain, a process called metastasis. No one dies from breast cancer that is confined to the breast.

- Median survival after a metastatic breast cancer diagnosis is three years. Median survival in 1970 was eighteen months. Men represent 1 percent of the deaths from metastatic breast cancer (410 deaths in 2012). About half a million deaths worldwide annually. [WHO]

- Incidence* Rates—one in eight women will be diagnosed with breast cancer. It's the second leading cause of death in women, exceeded only by lung cancer. After increasing for more than two decades, female breast cancer incidence rates began decreasing in 2000, then dropped by about 7 percent from 2002 to 2003.

- This large decrease was thought to be due to the decline in use of hormone therapy after menopause that occurred after the results of the Women's Health Initiative were published in 2002. This study linked the use of hormone therapy to an increased risk of breast cancer and heart diseases. Incidence rates have been stable in recent years. In the US, a woman is diagnosed with breast cancer every three minutes. One in eight women will have a diagnosis of breast cancer at some time in their life.

- Gender—226,870 women and 2190 men in the US in 2012 for a total of 229,060. Breast cancer is the most common cancer in women worldwide. It is also the principal cause of death from cancer among women globally. [WHO]

- Race—Compared to white women, African-American women are diagnosed at a higher rate under age forty and are more likely to die from breast cancer at every age.

- *Incidence is the number of newly diagnosed cases in a given year.*

- Young Women—Breast cancer is the number one cause of cancer death in young women under age fifty. Although breast cancer is often described as a *disease of aging*, 16 percent of the breast cancer deaths in 2012 were in this age group.

- Metastatic Research Funding—Estimated to be around 5 percent in Europe and less than that in US (2–3 percent) for metastatic research for *all* cancers.

- Time, money, and research needed to bring a new drug to market—On average, it takes eight to ten years and approximately $1 billion for a new drug to go from a chemistry model to FDA approval. Overall only 11 percent of drugs that start in clinical trials are eventually approved, but 34 percent of Phase 3 clinical trial drugs are approved. Every advance in breast cancer treatment and care has been the result of a clinical trial.

- It is still not known how to prevent recurrence or metastasis for most women, or how many of the women reported to have survived five years will go on to have a recurrence, but 30% will metastasize.

Sources:

ACS Breast Cancer Facts & Figures

American Cancer Society statistics 2000–2011

European Journal of Cancer 46 (2010) 1177–1180

NBCC—National Breast Cancer Coalition website

NCI SEER data analysis 2000–2005

O'Shaughnessy, "Extending Survival with Chemotherapy in MBC" The Oncologist 2005:10

Steeg, Patricia and Sleeman, Jonathan. "Cancer metastasis as a therapeutic target" Susan Love Research Foundation, 2015

World Health Organization

*Carol and Gene*

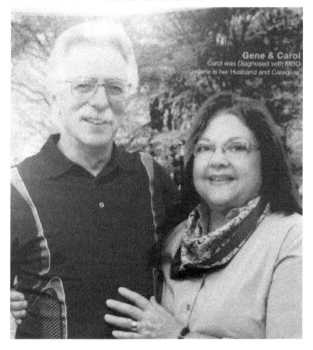

*Life is short, break the rules.*
*Forgive quickly, kiss slowly.*
*Love truly. Laugh uncontrollably and,*
*Never regret anything that makes you smile.*

—Mark Twain, American Writer

# BIBLIOGRAPHY

Cappello, Nancy M. PhD, Director and Founder, Are You Dense, Inc., State Density Reporting Laws, *www.areyoudense.org*, 2015.

Clark, Josh. *Why Is Mesopotamia Called the Cradle of Civilzation,* www. howstuffworks.com/history, 2014.

Daniels, Les. *The Golden Age of Wonder Woman.* Chronicle Books, San Francisco, CA, 2001.

Katze, Nicole. MA, Editor and Manager, *Living Alongside Cancer: The Power We Bring*, Publications, Living Beyond Breast Cancer, Insight, Fall, 2014.

Kubler-Ross, Elizabeth. *On Death and Dying.* Macmillan, London, England, 1969.

Lepore, Jill. *The Secret History of Wonder Woman.* Knopf, NY, 2014.

Steinem, Gloria and Chesler, Phyllis. *Wonder Woman,* A MS Book. Holt, Rinehart and Winston and Warner Books, NY, 1972.

Wilson, Robert A. MD, *Feminine Forever,* 3rd edition. W. H. Allen, London, England, 1966.

_____ Acts 17:26, the Bible, NIV.

_____ John 14:6, the Bible, NIV.

CPSIA information can be obtained
at www.ICGtesting.com
Printed in the USA
BVHW071137240521
607998BV00004B/423

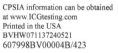

9 781637 671368